My Second Life

Living With Parkinson's Disease

Bill Harshaw

Introduction By Dr. C. David Naylor

16

EasyRead Large

9781525257292

RHYW

Copyright Page from the Original Book

Publisher: Anthony Hawke
Design: Jennifer Scott
Printer: Webcom

Canadian Cataloguing in Publication Data

Harshaw, William A. (William Archibald), 1943-
My second life: living with Parkinson's disease

Includes bibliographical references.
ISBN 0-88882-236-7

1. Harshaw, William A. (William Archibald), 1943- Health.
2. Parkinson's disease — Patients — Canada — Biography. I. Title.

RC382.H36 2001 362.1'96833'0092 C2001-930613-X

1 2 3 4 5 05 04 03 02 01

THE CANADA COUNCIL FOR THE ARTS SINCE 1957 | LE CONSEIL DES ARTS DU CANADA DEPUIS 1957

Canada

ONTARIO ARTS COUNCIL
CONSEIL DES ARTS DE L'ONTARIO

We acknowledge the support of the **Canada Council for the Arts** and the **Ontario Arts Council** for our publishing program. We also acknowledge the financial support of the **Government of Canada** through the **Book Publishing Industry Development Program, The Association for the Export of Canadian Books**, and the **Government of Ontario** through the **Ontario Book Publishers Tax Credit** program.

Care has been taken to trace the ownership of copyright material used in this book. The author and the publisher welcome any information enabling them to rectify any references or credit in subsequent editions.

J. Kirk Howard, President

Printed and bound in Canada.

Printed on recycled paper.

Dundurn Press
8 Market Street
Suite 200
Toronto, Ontario, Canada
M5E 1M6

Dundurn Press
73 Lime Walk
Headington, Oxford,
England
OX3 7AD

Dundurn Press
2250 Military Road
Tonawanda NY
U.S.A. 14150

TABLE OF CONTENTS

DEDICATION

My Second Life is dedicated to Dr. Tony Lang and Mrs. Jan Duff, RN, who have had a transforming influence on me. Without them I would not have had a second chance at life. They exercised the skills of their vocation with the ease of virtuosi and the passion of ones who care.

Words, endless words I've said to serve the moment—now it makes me proud to tell the truth.—Aeschylus

FOREWORD

by Dr. C. David Naylor

My Second Life is a remarkable and very personal account of one man's struggle with Parkinson's disease. Bill Harshaw's story is by turns poignant, gripping, sorrowful, irreverent, and—in the final analysis—uplifting.

On the one side, we have Mr. Harshaw—a highly intelligent individual with an indomitable spirit and a wickedly irrepressible sense of humour. This is a man who undergoes experimental brain surgery not once, but twice; and who, while coping with a disabling illness, lays out the design for what becomes Ontario's Trillium Drug Plan.

On the other side, we have the inexorable progression of the disease itself. Consider, for example, what one might expect to see upon encountering a person with moderately severe Parkinson's disease. Tremor is one of the manifestations that first brings Parkinsonism to the attention of the afflicted individual and his or her family. It is sometimes termed a "pill rolling tremor" because the movement of the thumb and forefinger resembles that which might be seen if the patient were rolling a tablet between his or her fingers. Loss of normal arm swing on walking is also common—this was one of the first manifestations of the condition in Bill Harshaw's case. As the disease progresses, the afflicted individuals develop a "mask-like" face with reduced blink frequency. (Canadians who last year watched television tributes to the late Pierre Trudeau may well have seen the dramatic change in the former prime minister's facial expressivity through the years as the disease exacted its toll on his nervous system.) The Parkinsonian's speech is gradually reduced in volume and clarity. Some will stammer at the start of sentences owing to difficulty co-ordinating the tongue, jaw, and lip motions required for normal articulation. Truncal rigidity will also be evident: rather than turning the neck or shoulders fluidly from side to side, Parskinsonians tend to move "en bloc." As the disease worsens, the patient's gait may degenerate into small shuffling steps. Gradually the Parkinsonian's ability to initiate and control movement of their limbs is impaired until they are more or less the prisoner of a rigid, trembling, unresponsive body. It is this latter phase that led London physician James Parkinson to characterize the disease as "paralysis agitans" in his classic "Essay on the Shaking Palsy" published in 1817.

In some ways, Alzheimer's disease is even more devastating, because it erodes the higher cortical functions that define us as human, leaving individuals who are shells of themselves. But as Alzheimer's disease progresses, its victims lose insight into their diminished mental capacity. Parkinson's disease is soul-destroying in quite a different way. Comparatively few Parkinsonians suffer cognitive impairment. The result is that most Parkinsonians are fully aware of their deteriorating physical function. Parkinson's in this respect resembles Lou Gehrig's disease—both these neurodegenerative conditions lead to progressive motor disability, leaving their victims mentally intact but alienated from their bodies.

The progression of Parkinson's is more vividly captured in *My Second Life* than in any other account I have read. By 1993, aged only 50, Bill Harshaw was immobilized for half a day and could otherwise move only with the aid of two walking sticks. Whenever he increased the doses of his anti-Parkinson's medications, he suffered intolerable side effects. When he reduced the doses he was simply unable to move. The challenges of coping with Parkinson's were compounded when Bill's beloved wife Esther was stricken with multiple sclerosis. Their independence was critically dependent on an amelioration of his symptoms and an improvement in his motor function. It was this desperate situation that led Bill Harshaw to undergo two different modes of experimental brain surgery, both performed of necessity with the patient wide awake. The extraordinary recovery of Bill's motor functions following surgery highlights the great potential of surgical palliation of this disorder.

But palliation it is—a reprieve of uncertain duration, with variable efficacy. For example, Bill's facial mobility remains reduced, and he continues to suffer from impaired speech. His handwriting, by his own description, is "hopeless," and he fatigues easily. More than a few of our telephone conversations have been exercises in mutual frustration. They are usually followed up promptly by an e-mail from Bill in which he makes his arguments in the same lucidly persuasive prose that enlivens this book.

While this is very much Bill Harshaw's story, I take some vicarious pride in the role played in this account by two of my colleagues who are world leaders in the field of Parkinson's disease. Both are based at the Toronto Western Hospital: Professor Anthony E. Lang holds the Jack Clark Chair in Parkinson's disease and Professor Andres M. Lozano is the Ronald Tasker Chair in Functional Neurosurgery at the University of Toronto. Even the names associated with these endowed chairs are part of the story of Parkinson's disease in Canada. Dr. Jack Clark, a prominent Canadian businessman, is a Parkinsonian who, together with his wonderful wife Mary, has been a tireless fundraiser for Parkinson's research. Dr. Ron Tasker is Professor Lozano's mentor and a pioneer in functional neurosurgery; he also assisted in the two operations on Bill Harshaw.

Bill's account will leave his readers in no doubt about the burden of living with Parkinson's for one courageous and unusual individual. But what may not be clear is just how burdensome Parkinson's is from a societal standpoint. We typically think of Parkinson's as "an old person's disease." That stereotype has been dispelled in part by the highly publicized case of the Canadian actor, Michael J. Fox. Bill Harshaw, for one, first noticed the symptoms of Parkinson's disease when he was only thirty-seven years old. It is true that more than 90 percent of all individuals living with Parkinson's disease are age 60 and over. But in a world where too many citizens work too hard and too fast, I believe it is no longer tenable to view diseases as less important if they preferentially destroy our well-earned leisure years rather than those decades in which we are harnessed to some occupation or another. As well, this condition does more than sap the quality of life of those afflicted. Despite modern drug therapy, Parksinsonism continues to be associated with sharply increased mortality.

All this might be less concerning if Parkinson's disease were extremely rare. It is not. Tens of thousands of Canadians are afflicted. The precise prevalence in this country is still unclear, but it is likely that at least three out of every one thousand adults in Canada suffers from some form of Parkinsonism. And, on a global basis, with population aging and the emergence of chronic, non-communicable diseases across developing countries, it is overwhelmingly probable that the burden of Parkinson's disease and related conditions worldwide will grow rapidly over the next several decades. It remains unclear whether the overall incidence of Parkinson's disease is rising independent of increases driven by population aging, the shifting burden of disease in developing countries, and improvements in survival. For that matter, we still do not understand exactly what causes the vast majority of cases of Parkinsonism. Medical science terms these cases "idiopathic"—a fancy way of acknowledging (or disguising) our continuing ignorance.

My Second Life is therefore more than Bill Harshaw's inspiring story. In my view, it is also a call to arms for funding agencies, philanthropists, and researchers alike. We simply know too little about Parkinson's disease. Our treatments are only modestly effective and essentially palliative. Some who are afflicted will—like Bill Harshaw—do reasonably well through sheer force of character, excellent medical care, and good fortune. For others, the disease advances at a mercifully slow pace. But for too many, Parkinson's disease imposes a relentless and progressive burden on their quality of life, culminating in a premature death. Bill Harshaw has written a book that will help a wide readership understand for the first time what it is like to live with Parkinson's. Now it is up to all of us to get on with finding a cure.

David Naylor, MD, DPhil, FRCPC
Dean, Faculty of Medicine
The University of Toronto

Perhaps you saw me. I was walking along Yonge Street in Toronto one day in the summer of 1993. Some passers-by would give me an unusual look, some a frightened, uncertain stare; a few even crossed over to the other side of the street. They were reacting to the contortions of my upper body. I was writhing uncontrollably, like some sort of primitive reptile and my face was distorted, mask-like. My walking was distinctly irregular, with both legs limping and dragging and I seemed almost incapacitated. I looked like an escapee from Wanless's freak show, which Robertson Davies so effectively described in his novel, World of Wonders.*My speech was blurred as if I was drunk. To people who encountered me I seemed to be incomprehensible, probably a lunatic, possibly dangerous.*

CHAPTER ONE

Outward and Visible Signs

In the summer of 1980 I thought the world was my oyster. I was thirty-seven. I had an exciting and challenging senior position as the treasurer of The Molson Companies Limited, one of Canada's oldest and most famous businesses. I was married to a loving and interesting wife, and we had two wonderful children. We lived in a pleasant house in north Toronto. We had a full social life and were active in the community and in the church and in politics.

My life was busy and satisfying, but it was often stressful. Every day I drove to work from our house in North Toronto to the Molson offices near the Toronto international airport. Much of the trip was along the 401, the multi-lane highway that bisects Metropolitan Toronto. The 401 is heavily traveled, indeed over-traveled and it is commonplace to witness accidents, some minor, and others horrendous. Often these cause the traffic to gridlock as emergency vehicles clear away torn heaps of metal and mangled humanity and other drivers pause to gawk at the carnage.

For me, this drive added stress and anxiety to the beginning and end of any working day, and now I was finding that sometimes it would leave me literally shaking. If the traffic was light and accident-free, I was fine. I did not bother telling Esther, my wife. Not much escapes Esther; she noticed the shaking too, but put it down to stress on the job. She did not even raise the subject. She became increasingly concerned when I would arrive home in the evening so exhausted that I could not even say "Hi" or "How are you." I had to recharge my batteries before I had the energy to greet our children and hear anecdotes from their day, or to pet our three-year-old Airedale terrier, Sir, who always greeted me eagerly at the door.

Esther had also begun to observe that my driving was becoming erratic, and that I was developing a tendency to oversteer to the right. She mentioned it often, telling me that I had better pay attention to my driving and stop woolgathering.

But now it was happening more often. Esther was afraid that I would have an accident and persistently questioned my driving ability. And when I was driving home one day that summer an accident did happen. It was not serious. There were no injuries, just a dent in my left front fender. The driver of the other car, which was in front of me, had tried to brake on wet pavement, skidded and spun around 360-degrees. Luckily I barely touched his car. The police constable on the scene gave me what seemed like a long lecture on the hazards of driving on the 401 and charged me with "following too closely." I was able to drive on, but when I got out of the car at home, I shook for half an hour. I didn't tell Esther.

I didn't feel like going to a friend's birthday party that night, but I went. I had a good time, but drank too much. I put it all down to stress.

But, from that moment on, I began to wonder. Was Esther right? Was my driving less than perfect? I did tend to over-steer. Still, I did not think anything was wrong with me that paying more attention to the road and developing better driving habits would not cure.

Esther's concern was born of love; I was foolish to have ignored it.

I had first noticed Esther Clark in Winnipeg on New Year's Day, 1967. I had gone with my father to the annual New Year's Day levée of the Archbishop of Rupert's Land at the See House, his official residence. Archbishop Clark was also the Primate—the head—of the Anglican Church of Canada. The levée, an open-house reception, was a full dress occasion. The military types were wearing their parade dress uniforms, the civilian men were in their morning coats, if they had them, ladies wore hats and gloves and The Most Reverend Howard Clark was attired in the court dress for a bishop—frock coat and gaiters, and patent leather shoes with silver buckles. He looked the part, except for an impish twinkle in his eyes that was most unepiscopal. There was an aura about the Archbishop, and he was obviously enjoying himself.

I was immediately attracted to Esther, one of his daughters. I told her I was thinking of going to a movie that afternoon. She responded with a chilly "enjoy yourself" that left me in no doubt that I would be going alone. I was certainly was not included in the group of friends who were invited to go upstairs to the library for "coffee," laced with rum, after the formalities.

I persisted. On an evening three months later, in March, 1967, I told Esther that I loved her. She said "don't," and left Winnipeg the next day. I lay siege to her at long distance, my weapon being a single red rose sent each week to her apartment in Toronto. Esther finally succumbed when a rose bloomed instead of dying on the spot. Changing florists proved to be a strategic move! On April Fool's Day, 1968, we became engaged.

It was July when I next saw the Clark family. I was invited to stay at their family cottage at Blue Sea Lake in the Gatineau hills. Mrs. Clark met me in Ottawa. As she drove—Coke in one hand, ice cream cone in the other and a box of Crackerjack wedged precariously between her knees—she pointed out the beauty of the Gatineau Valley and various landmarks *en route.*

In addition to her idiosyncratic driving, Mrs. Clark had a hostile relationship with snakes. On my first morning at Blue Sea, she cornered a garter snake and was about to kill it. She shouted, "Bill, get me an axe!"

"Don't you dare, Bill, or I'll never see you again!" yelled Esther from her second-floor bedroom, which was just above us. She then dashed down and out of the cottage and tussled with her mother. The snake escaped.

Later that day I noticed for the first time that the Archbishop had a fused back. "It must be very inconvenient not being able to move your neck" I observed tritely.

"Oh, not at all, Bill," he gracefully responded. "It makes swimming on my back so much easier." Howard Clark seemed an attractive but enigmatic man to me, and I was intrigued to see the Primate of the Anglican Church of Canada playing bridge, reading a Dorothy Sayers detective story and commenting on politics, sometimes all at once.

Our wedding had to be fitted in the Archbishop's tight schedule. He had been able to offer Labour Day, September 2, 1968. The wedding took place at St. George's-by-the-Lake, the little church near the Clark's cottage. It was an idyllic setting. Sandra Gwyn, in her book, *Tapestry of War,* describes Blue Sea as

> one of the loveliest and most lustrous of all the lakes in Gatineau country; more than twenty miles long, fringed with cedars and silver birches, framed by gentle, unintimidating mountains, dotted with islets and patches of water lilies.[1]

Esther was brought to the Church by her brother in a canoe. She sat on a high wooden armchair, wearing her grandmother's wedding dress, looking absolutely spectacular. There was a rain-shower during the service. As the service ended, so too did the shower, and a beautiful rainbow appeared in the window over the altar. We took this to be a portent of a long and fruitful, though not dull, marriage. Some commented that the rainbow was a sign from God that all tribulation was ended (Genesis, 9:13).

After we were married, we spent every July with the Clarks at Blue Sea Lake. Invariably we would play a rubber of bridge in the evening. One night, the Archbishop showed that he had his limits. Mrs. Clark had committed two sins—bidding improperly and getting the cards greasy by eating popcorn. Then Esther began recounting why she did not like part of John Updike's *Couples,* mainly the coarse language and graphic descriptions such as "this teenage boy was masturbating, and the semen came out with such force that it hit the light bulb on the ceiling, and shattered it."

"That does it!" said the Archbishop. He laid his cards on the table and left the room with a bemused look of exasperation.

Blue Sea became special to me, so much so that I abandoned my own family cottage near Kenora on Lake of the Woods. It had been the scene of too many unhappy memories. I had grown up there, but never enjoyed it because my father's endless work projects had made it resemble a labour camp more than a place for summer fun.

Esther and I started our married life in Winnipeg, but left after a few months when I received a good job offer from a subsidiary of Citibank in Toronto. I had started work in the investment business in Winnipeg on graduating from the University of Manitoba in 1965. I changed jobs three times. On each occasion the new company had sought me out and offered me a better job with more scope and challenge than the previous one had. The move to Toronto was an exciting opportunity for me.

I had worked hard for what I achieved and it was worth it. But putting myself on the fast track in the business world put me at odds with my father, whose modest career as a bank manger had left him embittered and resentful. While he would always say he was proud of my achievements, the compliments were usually backhanded and somewhat demeaning. My relationship with my parents, particularly my father, which was never very happy, had been deteriorating and I was glad to put some distance between us.

Later, in Toronto, when Citibank underwent a reorganization and I needed to find a new job, my father's often-repeated comment was, "I could have told you that would happen." I then moved to a good position at Wood Gundy, the investment house. It was a very positive career move, but it put me among the money changers in the temple as far as my father was concerned and set him against his oldest brother, my uncle Arch, who had had a much more successful business career and thought the move was a good one.

The move to Molson's came seven years later. One day, a Friday in July 1976, I answered the phone at about 4:30 in the afternoon. "Bill? Its Drew McCaughey at Molson. Our treasurer has jumped ship and gone to Weston's. I'd like you to join us as our treasurer. Are you still there? Good. Are you interested? Come over to the Yacht Club on the 1:45 boat on Sunday and we'll discuss it."

This was just about the highest compliment possible in the investment business. In the mid-seventies, it was rare for an investment professionals to be plucked from the analytical ranks of the brokerage industry. The job as treasurer of The Molson Companies Limited was a real coup. I was only 33 when I accepted the job, I had no corporate experience, and I was not a chartered accountant. I went to Molson in the fall of 1976. It was a job I loved. To be treasurer of Canada's oldest major family-controlled company was an honour any young executive would cherish. The job content was exciting too, with much of it new to me: commercial paper, managing the sinking fund, financing corporate growth, and being part of the team that worked on acquisitions and divestitures.

Shortly after we had arrived in Toronto, Esther became pregnant with our first child. It was a difficult pregnancy—through much of it she was confined to bed. It was a baby that was never meant to be, Esther later thought. The baby, a girl, was born on December 31, 1969, but the birth was complicated by a full breech presentation. She had a hairline fracture of the skull caused by the use of forceps and consequent internal bleeding. The doctors at the Wellesley Hospital advised transferring the baby to the Sick Children's Hospital. I accompanied our baby daughter in a taxi, the baby in an incubator, both of us supervised by a nurse. The prognosis was that if the baby should live, there would likely be severe brain damage and physical handicaps. Esther and I decided that we did not want medical science to make the supreme effort. We would let nature take its course.

I spent that night at the home of Esther's sister and her husband, Mary and Tony van Straubenzee, much of it by myself in a third floor bedroom crying.

Early on New Year's Day, 1970, I baptized our daughter "Megan Emily," using the words from *The Book of Common Prayer.* She died about half an hour later. Esther and I buried her ashes the next summer in the family plot in Napanee, without a clergyman present.

With our baby daughter's death we buried dreams of the future, not memories of the past. We were devastated by the death of Megan, but did not allow it to stop our efforts at starting a family. Our son Howard was born on May 14, 1971 and our daughter Emily on March 14, 1974. The sorrow and grief that was associated with that first pregnancy gave way to joy and hope fulfilled.

Our life was happy and hectic. I was a Churchwarden at Christ Church Deer Park, Esther was involved in the Anglican Church Women, and we were both involved in Progressive Conservative Party politics. Esther also ran the After Four programme at Davisville School. This activity was a natural outgrowth of her interest in arts and crafts—she did demonstrations of gingerbread houses and Easter egg decorating at Harbourfront each year. The *chef d'oeuvres* of her creative work were two large needlepoints after Wassily Kandinsky and Pablo Picasso.

Esther was her father's daughter. Bright and witty, fun at a party and intellectually very curious, she would, like her father, have four books going at once, on topics as varied as philosophy, eighteenth century literature, and psychology—the last-named was due to the career interest acquired when she was a probation officer—and a detective story thrown in for good measure.

Our friends reflected our interests—politics, the church—and were professional couples. Christ Church Deer Park is a special place to us. In the heart of midtown Toronto, this prosperous Anglican parish is where we have met many of our closest friends. There was just the right personal chemistry there. Stephen Booth was the Curate in 1971–74; he remains among my closest friends. Stephen is responsible, along with my father-in-law, for stimulating my intellectual development and encouraging me to think. I was a late bloomer. I now looked forward to the beginning of each day, because it was sure to be interesting and fun.

In the summer of 1980, things were going well at Molson, but there were some interesting business challenges. The company had been on a major acquisition programme since 1971, having acquired Beaver Lumber, a do-it-yourself retailer, and Diversey Corporation, a specialty chemical company. Meanwhile, a planned divestiture programme—selling off unwanted businesses—did not raise as much money as was planned for and what money was raised came in more slowly than our budget estimates. Then, in 1978, two major, unplanned acquisitions were made: the specialty cleaning chemical business of BASF Wyandotte and Le Club de Hockey Canadien—the famous Montreal Canadiens hockey team. This was at the time of the expansion of the National Hockey League. Molson was determined to maintain its premier marketing position on Hockey Night in Canada, a decision that was very expensive as it necessitated a substantial investment in advertising and promotional rights of the new expansion teams, Vancouver, Calgary, Edmonton, Winnipeg, and Quebec City. All this added up to a major cash shortfall for Molson's and a consequent increase in short-term borrowing.

Part of my job as treasurer was to devise funding strategy. I had proposed to the Board, and received authorization, for a major long-term financing. In addition I was in charge of the project team. It was a real feather in my cap. The financing was an issue of seventy-five million dollars of convertible debentures.

The project was progressing well, and we kept to our timetable but the prospectus work was demanding and the hours were long and sometimes when I got home after the drive along the 401 I was shaking with exhaustion and stress. I was undoubtedly working under some kind of handicap but it was not one I could identify or even recognize in myself.

Then one day that summer, I think it was in early August, after the preliminary prospectus had been filed, a senior vice-president who was a relatively new employee of Molson arrived in the middle of a meeting. It was the first interest he had shown in the issue. After taking a few minutes to orient himself, his opening comment rebutted a point I had been making.

"You are full of shit, Harshaw," he said in a grating English accent, and then proceeded to make his point. It was a dramatic opening and completely at odds with the tone of the meeting. Not to be outdone, I responded instantly, my tongue getting the better of me, as it often does: "I may be full of shit, but you are wrong. If you cannot make a useful contribution to this meeting, I will have to ask you to leave."

The tension could have been cut with a knife. Exchanges like that were rare at Molson. In a meeting with underwriters, and two sets of lawyers, they were unheard of. The vice president, very antagonistic, slammed shut his briefcase, got up and strode from the room, closing the door behind him with such violence that we were sure it must be damaged.

By common consent, it was agreed that I was in the right and the vice president's behaviour had been intolerable. The only problem was that he outranked me by two levels. As things turned out, my manager and mentor, who had brought me into Molson, left the company a few weeks later; the vice president was now my new manager. In December he, in effect, fired me. The execrable exchange between us was not referred to. I was given nine months to find a new job.

Esther did not view this turn of events as a tragedy, as I did, but as an opportunity. She knew I had always regretted not having taken law at university. Here was an ideal opportunity to take a few years off from corporate life and pursue that interest. She said, "So what if we have to scrimp for a few years? It will be worth it to see you with a job you're happy with." I had particularly felt the inadequacy during the acquisition and divestiture phase of my work at

Molson when the lawyers seemed to have much more influence. Alternatively, I could go back to the investment industry in the corporate finance side of the business. Or do both.

While I worked out my nine months at Molson, I entered a period that included grief, guilt, inadequacy, secrecy, and stupidity. These are all natural reactions to being fired; their intensity waxed and waned with the job prospects. The first few months were introspective, followed by alternating periods of optimism and pessimism as job interviews were lined up, and then did not pan out. I made a few short lists, but nothing went as far as an offer. This surprised me as I had been doing a good job at Molson; the problem had arisen due to a clash of personalities, not job performance.

Words of my father came back to haunt me. When I had first told him that I was considering leaving Wood Gundy to join Molson, he thought I must have been fired. He wouldn't believe that Wood Gundy took the Molson offer as a compliment. That is when he said: "You will fail, and when you do, by Christ, I hope you fall so hard that you can't get up." They were prophetic words, but hardly comforting.

Esther and I did not stop entertaining. We were known for having parties that were lots of fun with interesting people. I didn't lose my love of fun or my gregariousness. The big one that spring was a surprise party for Esther's fortieth birthday. I had invited fifty people, all of whom came. The party began at 6 in the evening and the last guest left at 2:30 in the morning.

My driving was still nerve-wracking. It was not getting worse, but neither was it improving as I'd hoped.

Then in the spring of 1981, Howard, who was now 10, was out jogging with me. I was a sporadic jogger and would take it up occasionally to try and lose weight and limber up. Howie said, "Dad, you must have really hurt yourself when you fell skiing last winter. Your right arm's not swinging." I paid no attention to his observation. After all, it didn't hurt.

In May and June Howard and I went on two canoe trips, one to Poker Lake in Haliburton with Stephen Booth, and the second to Algonquin Park with Tony Graham and his son Mark. Stephen and Tony are my closest friends, yet on neither excursion did I mention my limp arm or the fact that I was out looking for a job. This privacy—or secrecy, if you will, was singularly inappropriate. Tony, a doctor, is the Chief of Cardiology at the Wellesley Hospital in Toronto and Stephen, an Anglican priest, was himself in the middle of a combination job hunt and marriage break-up. I should have sought their advice and counsel instead of keeping quiet and feeling sorry for myself.

By the early fall of 1981, not long before I was due to leave Molson, a slight but perceptible tremor developed in my right arm.

I was not very easy to live with while all this was going on. I felt under a lot of pressure with the prospect of not having a job when my time ran out and increased worry about these damned symptoms of I didn't know what. To Esther I said, "I'm drinking more than usual—it's the stress of not finding a job." Through all this period, Esther was as loving and supportive of me as I could ever want. While trying to keep me on the straight and narrow, which wasn't the easiest thing to do, Esther consistently came up with good ideas. Her attitude was always positive, even if her patience was a bit short at times!

"Drinking is one of the stupidest things you can do," she said. "Supposing you had an accident when you've had too much. Or, what if you have a job interview and the tremor is there? They'd think you were hungover! Besides, you can't afford it. Smarten up! Stop drinking at lunch."

It was true, I was drinking at lunch, with a couple of fellows at the office. It was all on the expense account, so affording it wasn't an issue.

After my last day at Molson, September 30, 1981, there were tearful partings on my part, because this was the job I had loved, was proud of, and had been good at. Molson gave me an honourable settlement. Then I went out with my colleagues and wound up getting very drunk. We all did.

No job. I was getting desperate. The limp right arm persisted with a tremor, and I tried to conceal it by putting my hand in my trouser pocket, but then I feared I would be suspected of being a player of pocket pool. So, that was not a viable option. I must have tried every conceivable way of hiding my right hand—behind a chair, sitting on it, in my jacket in the Napoleonic style, behind my back ... the list could go on. The tremor was not so bad that people noticed it immediately, but if anyone looked carefully, there was no way to hide it.

Finally, in late October an offer came from Scotiabank. The offer was given in a most off-handed way. The executive who interviewed me said, "Well, you're not wearing Kodiaks or blue jeans; I guess you can have a job." No physical examination was required. It was not what I wanted and the pay was twenty percent less than I had been earning at Molson's, but it was a job. I took it, against Esther's advice, because I felt the obligation to support the family. It was a job I learned to hate.

Winter's treat was a limp in my right leg. I thought, "it's probably nothing, it will go away. It's all part of the stress of having to find a job." I told Esther and the children that I had tripped and fallen and twisted my ankle while jogging, and yes, I had hurt my shoulder when I was skiing the previous winter. I tried to ignore these problems: surely they would go away as I got settled in my new job, and that was just a matter of time. But still I wondered. Had the tremor been the reason why some companies never went beyond the first interview, or why some headhunters had not shortlisted me? Would Scotiabank fire me if it continued?

Esther was persistent. "Bill, there's more to it than twisting your ankle and hurting your shoulder last winter. These things are lasting too long. You have got to see Dr. Polak. It could be something serious." Jarda Polak had been our family doctor for several years.

Finally, I yielded to her unremitting pressure and arranged an appointment. On the day, I was apprehensive; scared shitless is a better, though less elegant expression. Why? It was fear of the unknown. I was all set to put the symptoms down to a hangover. We had been to a fund-raising dinner for David Crombie, then the Conservative Member of Parliament for Rosedale, the night before.

Dr. Polak did all the usual tests for a regular check-up.

When I mentioned the tremor, my arm not swinging and the slight limp, and tried to pass it off as the result of too much drinking, his interest picked up. He had me do a few tests that emphasized agility—touching my nose and then a moving pencil, opening and closing my hand and tapping my toes. Then he tested me with a sharp needle to see if there was feeling in every part of my body.

"There's more to this than occasionally drinking too much or the stress of looking for and adapting to a new job, Bill." But the usually very open Jarda Polak didn't give a hint of what he thought it might be.

The session finished very unsatisfactorily. He gave me no hint of what he thought was the problem. Instead, he said, "I'm going to refer you to Ron Macdonald. He's the Chief of Neurology at the Wellesley Hospital. He'll get to the bottom of this."

As I left, I was no further ahead than I was when I went in to his office. All I knew was that now I had to see a specialist. For what reason, I did not know. My apprehension was mounting.

Dr. Polak's secretary called a few days later with an appointment to see Dr. Macdonald in mid-February. I counted the days. At last, I would find out what was wrong with me, if anything.

CHAPTER TWO

Learning the Worst

It was a cold, blustery day in February, 1981. I found Dr. Macdonald's office in a wing of the Wellesley Hospital. It was a dismal building, a converted nurses' residence, dating from the 1940s. As I walked along the hallways I could see that some of the doctors had made the best of a bad thing by imaginatively decorating their offices and waiting and consultation rooms. Not Dr. Macdonald. His office had battleship linoleum on the on the floors and a depressing beige/taupe paint on the walls, unrelieved by any decoration at all.

Dr. Macdonald was an unremarkable man physically with an easy if impersonal manner. It took me a while to grasp that his very ordinary appearance concealed a very sharp mind, quick to pick up nuances and subtleties, and with a keenness for high technology.

By way of introduction he said, "You know, Bill, diagnosing neurological conditions is particularly difficult. It has to be done by inference because the brain cannot be examined directly. A brain biopsy—a small sample—cannot be taken and examined like other organs. For example, your tremor could be Parkinson's, multiple sclerosis, essential tremor, or progressive supra nuclear palsy—that last one's a killer. There are a few other neurological diseases that could also be a possibility, but they are so rare that it would be like looking for zebras rather than horses."

He took my history and asked, "Anyone in your family ever have any neurological conditions?"

Not knowing what they were, I asked, "Like what? One of my father's sisters had 'nerves.' Is that what you mean? They would never say what it was except 'nerves.'"

"That's an old-fashioned expression! Was she crazy?"

"Yes, very much so! She spent most of her life in a mental hospital."

"Bill, she was probably mentally ill, likely schizophrenic. I meant multiple sclerosis, that sort of thing."

I sort of vaguely knew. Esther's aunt, her mother's twin sister, after whom she'd been named, had multiple sclerosis for many years before she died. She had evidently been a wonderful, fun-loving woman whose husband's early death from a heart attack had turned her bitter. She had contracted MS later in life, and had great difficulty walking.

Dr. Macdonald then proceeded to the diagnosis. Methodically, but without telling me what he was looking for, he put me through a number of tests: opening and closing my fist, tapping thumb and index finger quickly, tapping toes and heels, walking, heel and toe, balancing on one foot, pinprick to test me for feeling, plus others I cannot remember. Many of them were the same tests Dr. Jarda Polak had done a few weeks earlier. When it was all over, he said in an emotionless voice, "Well, what did Jarda tell you he thought it was? He's usually pretty good at this."

"He didn't say"

"That's unlike him. You have Parkinson's disease, Bill. So far its only on your right side."

I felt as though I had been punched in the groin, and then I became nauseous. I thought I was going to lose control of my bladder and bowels for a few seconds, but I did not. I must have turned white as a sheet; I know I broke out in a sweat, because Macdonald handed me a damp towel before he continued, "Funny thing, Parkinson's. Don't know what causes it, don't have a cure for it either. And it doesn't progress at the same rate in everyone. So, in ten years time, you might be the same as now or two years from now you might be a quivering bowl of jelly."

Dr. Ronald Macdonald, the Chief of Neurology at the Wellesley Hospital in Toronto, had no hesitation in his voice, neither was there a hint of equivocation. He was like a judge delivering a verdict from which there is no appeal.

"Are there any tasks that you are finding either more difficult or impossible to perform?"

I said, "Just one thing. Tying flies for fly fishing and tying the fly onto the leader."

"We'll have you back to normal, tying those things on in no time," he said cheerily. "Parkinson's is very idiosyncratic in the way it strikes individuals. Some people have great problems tying shoe laces while others will have no trouble at all. Bring samples of your handwriting over the past two or three years to your next appointment. I want you to have a CAT-scan before you see me as well. It's new technology. It allows us to have a detailed look at the sections of your brain that may be affected. Much better than X-rays! It will be absolute confirmation that you have it."

I decided to walk part of the way home. I noticed my right eye was tearing involuntarily. What did Macdonald mean when he said it was on my right side only? Soon there were full-blown tears from both eyes. I must be a fine sight, I thought, looking like the derelicts that live and hang out around here. I walked from the Wellesley Hospital a few blocks to the Yonge-Bloor subway stop, wondering what I would tell Esther. Apart from the "bowl of jelly" comment, Macdonald hadn't told me what to expect from Parkinson's. Anyhow, the symptoms weren't that serious now. You had to be pretty observant to notice them. Or so I thought.

I remembered Granny Gwyn, my maternal grandmother, who had died in 1968. She had

Parkinson's, we were told. All she had was the tremor, and not all that badly. Then there was John Diefenbaker, the former prime minister of Canada, whose head shook and he had the tremor as well. That frightened me because I remembered the 1967 Tory party leadership convention and how paranoid Diefenbaker had seemed to me in that year.

Esther was just waking up from an afternoon nap when I got home from the hospital. She asked, "What did the doctor say was wrong with you?"

"Parkinson's disease, on my right side only," I said, trying to minimize the bad news.

Esther started sobbing. "What does this mean will happen to you? How does it get worse? What is the outlook?"

Not only had Macdonald not been very forthcoming in laying out the implications of Parkinson's in both the short and long term, I had not been very inquisitive in asking about them. We decided to do nothing until we saw Macdonald together. We had an appointment in about two weeks time.

In the meantime, I had a CAT-scan. It was a huge machine in the basement of the Wellesley Hospital. It took about half an hour to set up and "take the pictures." Part of me was still rejecting Macdonald's diagnosis. Surely there was some mistake. I was desperate for any glimmer of hope. A taciturn technician would only say, "Your doctor will tell you the results."

Esther had begun reading about Parkinson's and she and I went together to the next appointment with Dr. Macdonald. He wanted to ascertain the "progression" of my Parkinson's and we wanted to gain information.

Talk about a man happy in his job. Macdonald's enthusiasm and obvious pleasure in demonstrating his skill in making correct diagnoses of medical conditions that don't get better was a bit hard to take. It's one thing to enjoy your work; it's quite another to seem to take pleasure from giving bad news.

"Good thing you had the CAT-scan. No doubt about it now! Also your handwriting. You can see the deterioration over three years. That's confirmation too! It's very unusual for someone so young to get Parkinson's. You're the youngest patient I've had with it. I would guess that there aren't fifteen people under forty with Parkinson's in Ontario. We know approximately how quickly it will progress in a typical patient, one who's over sixty when diagnosed, but I have no experience with young onset. The worst cases wind up being immobilized because their arms and legs go rigid. But not everyone is a worst case. It is a very individual disease. Sorry I can't be more help."

If he knows that it's Parkinson's, perhaps he can do something about it, I thought.

"Are there any drugs I can take? What can I do about it?"

"Nothing for the time being, Bill. All I have established is that you have Parkinson's. This examination has given me your "baseline," against which I'll be able to measure your progress. Its a chronic progressive disease. What you would normally call "getting worse," we call "progress." Anyhow, I won't be prescribing any drugs until I can get an idea of the rate it's moving. It's not bad enough for drugs yet."

"That wasn't much help," I grumbled as we left.

"Now, Bill, he seems like a good man. They just don't know that much about Parkinson's," said Esther.

All we knew about Parkinson's was what Dr. Macdonald had told me and what Esther had read. It is a chronic degenerative disease of the brain. I got in touch with my closest medical friend, Tony Graham. His advice was to read up on the condition. The advice was good but the result depressing.

The books and pamphlets all seemed to stress the worst that could happen: the patient physically immobilized with the face an impassive mask, or minimally active, dependent on a friend or relative for day-to-day living. I quickly decided to avoid reading about Parkinson's. Esther hid the most depressing book from me. To this day I have not seen it. I was determined that I would never become like that. And the easiest way was to deny that I even had Parkinson's.

Esther read everything she could get her hands on. She would say to me after reading a book or article about Parkinson's, "Bill, this is fascinating. They're really making progress in finding out how the drugs get to the part of the brain where they can do the most good. That means that your drug dose can be lower because it won't be wasted."

"Big deal," I would huffily reply. "He won't even put me on any drugs yet. It's a waste of time."

I did read the classic description of Parkinson's. In 1817, twenty years before Queen Victoria ascended the British Throne, Dr. James Parkinson, a London physician and social activist, wrote his "Essay on the Shaking Palsy," which described six patients with a slowly progressive physical disease. All of them had the following characteristics:

> involuntary tremulous motion, with lessened muscular power, in parts not in action even when supported, with a propensity to bend the trunk forward and to pass from walking to a running stance.

It is an elegant piece of English prose: this description of Parkinson's disease has not been improved upon in the eighteen decades that have passed. And it was all I wanted to know. But inevitably I learned more.

I learned that the cause of Parkinson's has not been discovered, neither has a cure been found. Dr. Parkinson, in his essay, also noted that after a stroke, the characteristic tremor was less evident, although muscle weakness more than made up for the eased tremor. None of the medications or surgical procedures that have been developed over the years have cured the disease. Instead, they have purchased some of that elusive commodity called time and have allowed the patients to live more comfortably than they otherwise would have done. The condition progressively worsens, with the most advanced patients eventually immobilized.

Parkinson's disease results from the death of nerve cells at the base of the brain called the *substantia nigra,* literally "black substance." These cells produce two key brain chemicals, seratonin and dopamine, a neurotransmitter that brain cells use to communicate with each other. Without dopamine, the thought of lifting an arm can't be transferred into the act of lifting an arm. As the cells die, the production of dopamine slows down and the motor system begins to shut down. By the time a patient is diagnosed 80 percent of the *substantia nigra* cells are dead.

But it has not been discovered why the *substantia nigra* cells die: do they die fighting off Parkinson's, or as a result of Parkinson's?

I tried to persuade myself that if no one knew I had Parkinson's, then I didn't have it. I wanted to deny to myself and to the world-at-large that I had Parkinson's. Friends and acquaintances, with a few exceptions, weren't told by me, but by Esther. I didn't want to talk about it, but I was in the awkward position of not knowing who knew and who didn't. Early on, we told Esther's parents. Mrs. Clark's advice was not to tell anyone, particularly the bank where I worked. Her reasoning was that you don't tell the world about imperfections in your family. We decided, for the time being, to say nothing to the children about Parkinson's.

At the same time I was trying to deny having Parkinson's, I was very self-conscious of my appearance. By this time, anyone observing me closely would know something was wrong. There was the tremor in my arms, suggestive of the "morning-after shakes," the DTs that the comedian Shelley Berman so graphically described in his monologue "The Morning After the Night Before." There was also the dragging of my right foot, which I passed off as shin splints or tendonitis from running. I also realize now that Parkinson's (or the side effects of medications) was beginning to have an effect on my judgement. Concentration was not a problem but my ability to prioritize was affected.

Fly fishing is the one sport I love. It is unlike any other form of fishing. Delicacy and grace are its hallmarks. These qualities are precisely the ones that Parkinson's strikes. I was determined that I would not stop fishing. Stephen Booth was one of the very first people that I told about my diagnosis. He was my fly-fishing mentor and now helped me tie my flies to the leader—a task that called for more dexterity than I could manage. I cursed Macdonald for the breezy assurance he had given me in my first appointment that I would be back to normal. I had never been able to cast with the elegance of a really good fisherman like Stephen, so any deterioration here was probably marginal. It was my first conscious experience of making a trade off: accept a little help in order to do something you really enjoy. The price was a marginal loss of independence. It was well worth it.

At work, things were not going well. I began as a supervisor in Canadian Corporate Credit, with the understanding that once I picked up the bank's way of doing things, I would move over to Corporate Banking, the marketing arm, which was where the action was, and related more to my previous experience. For reasons that were never clear to me, that move never came.

Sometime in the fall of 1982, I had told my manager at the bank that I had Parkinson's. He reacted with indifference. "It's not a problem now. Let me know when it starts to affect your performance." I had built up telling him into such an important episode, that I felt really let down. I thought, it just goes to show that everyone is making a mountain out of a molehill about Parkinson's.

My first manager was, by the standards I had been previously accustomed to, detail-oriented and continually checking up on me. He was typical of middle managers in the bank. The bank was unlike any other place I had worked. Coming from Molson's, and indeed, from all my other jobs, the culture shock was serious. I had been used to setting my own priorities and working in an open environment. Now I had to get used to the way the bank was organized and managed. A financial and lending institution as large and geographically diverse as Scotiabank must be centralized. And centralized it was.

I was grappling with overlapping problems: learning to adjust to the bank's business culture, my new job and trying to deal with an uncongenial boss, and at the same time learning to cope with Parkinson's, while keeping it a secret from everyone who did not need to know. In retrospect, I realize what a tremendous mental strain it was trying to keep those balls in the air. I also now know that my biggest mistake was to keep Parkinson's a secret.

In the first place, I am not a good liar, and since you have to tell different stories to different people and remember them, the mental effort is colossal. The other consequence of secrecy and denial is that you eventually remove yourself from reality and live in a fantasy world. If the rest of the world perceived that something was wrong with me, I separated myself from everyone else by saying, "No, nothing is wrong with me. Your perception of me is incorrect." It doesn't take much imagination to see that this sort of behaviour, if carried out at the extreme, can be very dangerous.

To a limited degree, an element of denial may be healthy in order to avoid being preoccupied with the seemingly inevitable horror that Parkinson's offered. But, by removing yourself from reality, you live in a fantasy world, alienated from society. That is what denial does and, for a time, it did it to me.

My denial was based on a simple fatalism: the progress of Parkinson's was relentless and inevitable. If the cause was unknown and there was no cure, then why not just do nothing and ignore it. The problem with fatalism is that it breeds ideology; indeed it is an ideology. It was easy to be seduced by this simplistic approach to Parkinson's; conversely, it was hard not to be captivated, particularly as I hated my job. I thought, I will just stay put in my life. No one seemed to care, except Esther, and she was doing nothing but reading articles about Parkinson's. I think I ignored them because they offered some hope when, increasingly, I only wanted unremitting despair.

Meanwhile, Esther was ready to devote more time outside the home. She had developed a serious interest in public education and decided to run for school trustee in the municipal elections. One of the things that had spurred her on was when her mentor, David Crombie, the former mayor of Toronto, and later a federal MP, told her, "You will have more influence, and have a better chance of being a positive force for change at the School Board than a backbencher in Ottawa, or even a cabinet minister." On November 12, 1982 Esther was elected a public school trustee on the Toronto Board of Education. It gave her a new lease on life, just at the time I felt my lease had been cancelled. I enjoyed the excitement and activity of the campaign, but after it was over, life settled down to the drudgery of routine for me and the challenge of being a practising politician for Esther.

A few months later, in January 1983 Esther's father died, just three months short of his eightieth birthday. Neither Esther nor I realized at the time what a watershed event this would be in our lives. In the fifteen years that we had been married, I had developed a very warm affection and friendship for my father-in-law. The Archbishop—despite my close relationship to him I always called him Archbishop Clark or Your Grace—was kind and thoughtful. He helped me maintain a balance as my relationship with my father went from bad to worse. In the summer of 1980, he wrote in a letter to me: "I still don't understand what makes Jim Harshaw tick ... but a final break is very final and should be resorted to only after full opportunity has been allowed for the matter to die down."

I had not realized how close Esther had been to her father. For her, God died, or at least went into a coma, when her father died. Esther had set standards for herself that were unattainable. As long as her father was alive, this did not pose a problem, because the standards were based on him. But after his death she had great difficulty finding a balance between her ideals and what she could realistically attain.

In the fall of 1983, Dr. Macdonald started trying out some medications on me. I had been diagnosed for about eighteen months and was becoming increasingly frustrated. I was pretty testy at the now standard question from people, "What's wrong with your leg, Bill?" Acquaintances were frequently pointing out that I was no longer my usual jolly self. After one such observation, I said in frustration: "Goddammit, even Santa Claus isn't in a good mood all the time! Why should I be?" Secretly, during the long nights when I didn't sleep, the inevitable questions would come to mind: "Why me, God? What have I done to deserve this? It's a hell of a punishment. Was I that bad?" The answers were some time in coming, in fact they still are.

Every three months, I saw Dr. Macdonald and he prescribed pills that were mostly useless (Symmetral, for example) and, in one case, worse than useless. Cogentin was supposed to ease the tremor, but a side effect screwed up my vision so badly that new glasses were rendered useless in four months. I would throw my glasses on the floor in frustration. This would not be the only time the side effects of drugs proved to be intolerable. Finally, he put me on Sinemet, the major anti-Parkinsonian drug, which seemed to work.

It is not unusual for a Parkinson's patient to have adverse reactions to a medication. The possible side effects are usually discovered during the clinical trial phase of a drug and their existence is disclosed in product monographs so that all physicians can be aware of them before prescribing them. Many are no worse than an upset stomach for a few days, but some are very serious. For instance, L- dopa-based medications can cause hallucinations and other psychological reactions in patients. That is why neurologists are leery of prescribing regular doses at the beginning. Perhaps the reason for these adverse reactions is that the brain goes from a dopamine deficiency (characteristic of Parkinson's) to a dopamine surplus with various side effects. The majority of which are not serious—mild nausea, drowsiness, headaches—but some are intolerable.

L-dopa was first introduced in 1967. It revolutionized drug therapy for Parkinson's, replacing medications based on alcohol extracts from various herbs and plants, even from the deadly nightshade. The drug based on elixir of nightshade was supplemented by white wine, charcoal, bread dough, sawdust, and nutmeg. L-dopa was able to cross the blood-brain barrier and effectively replace some of the dopamine that had been lost. The adverse reaction that goes along with it is dyskinesia (literally "bad movement"): involuntary fragmentary, jerky or incomplete body motions. It can be mild, or extreme, taking up a radius of two and a half feet.

In the late winter of 1984, Dr. Macdonald said at what turned out to be my last appointment with him:

"I am referring you to Tony Lang at the Western. I refer all my difficult patients to him."

It is a measure of my paranoia that I felt abandoned, deserted. I recognized Dr. Macdonald was a good diagnostician even if his manner of relating to me wasn't the greatest. I trusted him and felt he was looking after me well. I knew I was a bit aggressive sometimes, but was I really all that difficult?

In fact, although I didn't realize it at the time, Dr. Macdonald was doing me the one of the greatest services a doctor can do: referring a patient whose care is beyond his ability to another specialist. His choice of words that day left something to be desired. What he meant was that my case of Parkinson's was difficult, not that I—Bill Harshaw—was difficult. But that was not what I understood at the time.

It was now three years after my initial diagnosis and the symptoms were very obvious. Parkinson's had advanced to my left side. Its progress was like a regiment on a slow march to the beat of its own drummer. I had tremors in both arms and I was dragging both feet. To those who asked, I would say the same sort of thing I had been saying for three years: "I sprained my ankle skiing", or "Damn jogging, gives me tendonitis!" Hiding my tremor was another matter. I used the old hangover excuse to anyone who asked.

One Sunday at church there was a visiting priest who told us during the coffee time after the service that he was on his way to an assignment in San Francisco. His behaviour seemed a bit off the wall, but Cranmer's phrase that the church should welcome "all sorts and conditions of men" presumably applied to the clergy as well as to lay people. He said to me "That shaking of your hands looks to me as though you did some pretty serious drinking last night. Do you have a drinking problem?"

My friends were shocked by his comment and the off-hand way he made it. We were not surprised when he turned out to be an imposter posing as an ordained priest.

I kept on exercising every day, cross-country-skiing in the winter and canoe tripping with Howard in the summer. On the canoeing expeditions, Howard increasingly carried the organizational load, and a larger part of the physical burden. It was sometimes hard on him, but there were no complaints. Esther had told him he was to take control.

I had to keep coming up with a positive answer for myself to the question: "Can I still do it, or does Parkinson's make a difference?" For about five years, until 1986, I kept on pretending that if it made a difference at all, it only slowed me down a bit. That was all there was to it! Most of the time I felt alright, or so I kept telling myself. A curious thing about Parkinson's, or at least my version of it, is that it is not a physically painful condition. I might be trembling or immobilized but no pain was associated with these conditions. Mental anguish was another matter.

One thing I did not do at this time was have anything to do with the Parkinson's Foundation, the organization established to provide support for Parkinsonians and their families and to raise money for research into Parkinson's. Having taken a fatalistic approach to my condition, when I wasn't denying it, I decided I didn't need any help from fellow sufferers. Besides, someone had said to me, "I wouldn't waste my time going there ... run by a group of well-meaning matrons ... meetings pretty depressing ... nothing worse than a group of Parkinsonians...." It was several years before I began to appreciate the value of the Foundation and the support it could offer.

Gradually I realized that I was seriously, chronically depressed, but I did not entirely know why. Dr. Macdonald had not picked up on this. Again, in retrospect, the reasons are obvious enough. The shock of being told I had a chronic progressive neurodegenerative disorder inevitably had negative implications, not only for my own quality of life but for the well-being of my family. Would I be fired from the bank for having Parkinson's? Was my job performance adversely affected by it? Were my compensation increases and promotion limited by Parkinson's? These all contributed to an external reasons for being depressed. But there was an internal or biological reasons as well.

The chemical balance of the brain is altered by Parkinson's because of the dopamine deficiency. This deficiency in itself leads to depression. So, I had two reasons to be depressed. Three, really: I hated my job.

It was very dangerous at work for me because Parkinson's was causing significant problems at work and my silence about it was a contributing factor. A departmental reorganization had taken place and I had a new manager. If my first manager had been a problem for me, my second was a disaster. We had a basic personality clash, and he was "on my case" from the first day. He was a Maritimer of modest background and similar ability, who had by dint of hard work and long hours progressed from being a Scotiaplan loan inspector in rural Nova Scotia—a quite big fish in a smallish pond—to a senior post in the bank's high profile Corporate Banking Division—a largish fish in a huge pond. But he was a small town boy at heart, and he was uncomfortable in Toronto; what is more, he deeply resented those who were at ease in the financial centre of Canada.

Stupidly, I had not told him about my Parkinson's. My first performance appraisal from him was as negative as it could possibly be, down in the "needs improvement" category. Everything from poor work to insubordination was mentioned. This was serious business.

Then to cap it off, he said to me, "About your drinking problem. I am arranging for you to attend The Donwoods Institute—a substance abuse treatment centre—so you can come to grips with the excessive drinking you do."

I was shocked. It is true I had drunk too much in my latter days at Molson's, but that was a thing of the past. For one thing, I no longer could afford to drink at lunch or after work—my salary at the bank was twenty percent lower than at Molson and the bank did not view social drinking as a business expense. For another, much of my youth had been spent coping with my father's drinking—he had been an alcoholic and I had the scars to show for it. I was determined that Howard and Emily would not have the miserable childhood I did. Howell Raines, in his book *Fly Fishing Through the Midlife Crisis* writes,

> Fortunate is the man who cleans up his act soon enough that his children's memories of him won't be fodder for their therapy sessions.[2]

My manager's comments made me feel helpless. It took me some time to realize that I was the author of my own misfortune. By not saying anything about Parkinson's at work, by actively denying I had any serious problems, I had set myself up for the worst of all possible worlds.

CHAPTER THREE

Coming Out

In May of 1984 I had my first appointment with Dr. Tony Lang at the Toronto Western Hospital's Movement Disorders Clinic. Lang's clinic was busy, and there was a sense of organized chaos about it. Somehow it seemed warm and friendly, and it reflected Sir William Osler's description of medicine as "a calling in which your heart will be exercised equally with your head." The "flow" was managed by Mrs. Jan Duff, RN, who gave life to another of Osler's aphorisms: "The trained nurse has become one of the great blessings of humanity."

Before the appointment I had been sent an exhaustive questionnaire to fill out. It seemed to cover all the medical information one could want to know for assessing a Parkinson's patient and then some. Dr. Lang told me that he wished all his patients took such care in filling out forms. He proceeded to ask questions arising from the questionnaire. I had great confidence in him. After completing the questionnaire and the interview, I felt I had transferred to Dr. Lang virtually all my knowledge of myself. He then called in one of his colleagues, described my symptoms, and asked what he would recommend. The other doctor responded with a suggestion to add to the medication

I had been taking. Lang commented, "My thoughts exactly."

He confirmed that I had Parkinson's. That was not as redundant as it might seem. There are several neurological conditions that have some symptoms in common, but are in fact quite different. Consequently, approximately one-quarter of all patients initially diagnosed with Parkinson's are later re-diagnosed with another condition. Other possibilities unrelated to Parkinson's, to name only two killers, were Shy-Dragger's Syndrome and Progressive Supra-Nuclear Palsy. Dr. Lang ruled these and then gave me the bad news.

Early onset patients, those who clearly have Parkinson's before the age of 50, have much more rapid symptom progression than do patients who develop the condition when they are older. "Not very pleasant," he said breezily, "but I think you should know this. Dr. Macdonald was right when he told you that Parkinson's is very individual, so I can't be specific about its rate of progress. You might begin considering the possibility that you will have to stop working long before your normal retirement age."

The news was not good. But I had been treated as an adult, capable of understanding the consequences of what he was saying. I went away with a new prescription in my pocket, this one for Bromocriptine, a dopamine agonist. There are dopamine transmitting cells and receiving cells, the latter being called receptors. An agonist is a drug that activates a dopamine receptor, extending length of time that the L-dopa medication remains active in the brain, like a catalyst. And at first it seemed to make me feel better.

I didn't realize that I was falling into the typical Parkinsonian's trap. Following on my assumption that Dr. Lang was omniscient as far as my case of Parkinson's was concerned, it was an easy leap to the expectation that every prescription and recommendation would be successful. I could not tell that, in some cases, I was experiencing the "placebo effect," the illusion of feeling better simply from being treated. That is why clinical trials of new drugs include "double blind" tests in which neither the physician nor the patient know if a particular patient is taking the real drug that is being tested or a placebo.

While I understood at an intellectual level what Dr. Lang was saying about the possible implications of Parkinson's for me, that abstract assessment did not spill over into concrete reality for a couple of years. I still was not ready to accept the fact that I had Parkinson's, and to consider the possible consequences for me and my family. I was almost schizophrenic in my attitude to Parkinson's. I could have an intellectual conversation about chronic illness or Parkinson's, but I would not consider my family in relation to my Parkinson's. As simple a thing as discussing the practical effects of Parkinson's with the children was not on my agenda. Howard, who was now 14, and

Emily, who was 11, knew I had Parkinson's, but were unaware, or so I thought, of the implications. In fact, as they observed my condition deteriorating, or, in the perverse language of medicine, progressing, they assumed the worst.

One evening Esther, who had been a school trustee for over two years by this time, had her assistant over for a family dinner. In the course of the evening he talked about an uncle of his who, he said, had died of Parkinson's. He went into a lot of grisly and, I felt, unnecessary detail. What killed him, the assistant said, was his inability to swallow. Apparently all the things that could go wrong in a Parkinsonian went wrong with the uncle and he choked to death on his own saliva. In the middle of his story our guest realized what he was saying and the effect it was having. With each attempt to extricate himself from this tale of horror, his foot became more deeply implanted in his mouth.

Howard and Emily were transfixed by this account of Parkinson's and the death it caused. Howard was egging him on. Each time the man paused, Howard, eager for more information, would say, "Go on!" Later that night, Emily was sitting on the chaise longue in our bedroom with tears streaming down her face. She wailed to Esther, "I'm watching Daddy die before my eyes—he's shaking to death!" It took some time to calm her down. She was convinced by the version of the reality of Parkinson's she had heard at dinner, because it was the only account of Parkinson's she had heard.

Up to that time I had said virtually nothing to either Howie or her, assuming in my passive-aggressive fashion that things would work out in the fullness of time, that there was no need to discuss Parkinson's because of the inevitability of it all. There was nothing I could do about Parkinson's, so why discuss it? Both children bottled up their concerns. Emily repressed them. That year, Howard went away to Sedbergh, a boarding school near Montebello, Quebec, and was not faced with the problem on a daily basis. We had not sent him away to school because of my Parkinson's but because we thought he would benefit from a change of environment. After some initial problems, his years at Sedbergh were a great success.

Nonetheless, everyone in the family except Esther was now actively involved in denial. The strain on all of us was immense, and it spilled over to episodes of anti-social behaviour for both children. They would each become very withdrawn, exploding from time to time when the pressure of denial got too great for them.

This put an incredible burden on Esther, whose focus was more inward than the children's. The difference was that she tended to implode, resulting in periods of depression that were almost disabling in their severity. Such was the effect of my denial. My family was becoming dysfunctional.

One weekend, Esther and I went to Sedbergh school for a parents' weekend. On the Saturday, after the interviews with the teachers were over, I went cross-country skiing with Howie and his friend and the friend's parents. I was lagging behind. When asked if I was having trouble, I replied: "damn shin splints are giving me a problem!" It was really Parkinson's of course, but I wasn't going to let my secret out to anyone who didn't have to know.

As I struggled with my denial of my Parkinson's and the reality of it, I often had difficulty squaring this experience with my Christian faith. Sometimes I thought of the phrase "an outward and visible sign," from the traditional Anglican definition of a sacrament. With Parkinson's it has always seemed to me a cruel irony, because the other half of the definition, "of an inward and spiritual grace" could not be further from the truth. Spiritual grace is "the supernatural assistance of God, bestowed upon a rational being, with a view to his sanctification." There was no grace associated with Parkinson's for me: if anything it was just the opposite. I was reminded of the lines from Archibald MacLeish's play, *J.B.*:

> I heard upon his dry dung heap
> That man cry out who cannot sleep:
> "If God is God He is not good,
> If God is good He is not God
> Take the even, take the odd, I would not sleep
> here if I could
> Except for the little green leaves in the wood

And the wind on the water.[3]

About this time I came across an article by Norman Cousins, a distinguished American journalist who had discovered his inner resilience to a chronic medical condition and captured it in a phrase: "defiance, not denial." By this he meant that if you accept a chronic illness, and even its inevitable progress, you can still defy it to have a negative mental effect on you, provided a sense of humour is retained. At this time, early 1985, I thought that Cousins was pretty facile and superficial. After all, what did he know? He was only a writer. It took me many years to realize the depth of his experience and to admire his ability to express it in clear, simple prose.

What he had done in a humanistic way, was to inject hope, the greatest of the Christian expectations, into a life with chronic medical conditions. For instance, as movement becomes more constrained, the patient should think "What things can I do now that I could not do before? How can I turn my constraints to advantage?"

But at this point in my life, I was not thinking of new freedoms or how I could profitably use the hours when Parkinson's left me immobile. I was far too busy feeling sorry for myself. I had a long way to go. I had no promises to keep, just miles to go before I slept.

I knew that Esther's father, Archbishop Clark, had succeeded brilliantly in turning disadvantage to advantage. When spondylitis forced him to take nine months off from his duties as Dean of Ottawa, Clark did not just languish in bed feeling sorry for himself. Instead, he used his time to great profit reading philosophy and theology as well as coming to know his five children better. Knowing that my father-in-law had made a success of his illness was not merely a part of the family's lore, it was part of the Anglican Church's. If that was not enough to put me off, I do not know what would be. It was so much easier to be a failure: no one expects anything of you! If I was not careful, I would wind up with a ruined family and a promising career cut short as my sole legacy.

The situation at the bank was tricky. At work, I was frightened. I'd put myself in a real pickle. By claiming being hungover as the reason for my tremor, I had set myself up for my manager to conclude that I had a drinking problem serious enough to warrant sending me to Donwoods to have it treated. My initial focus wasn't on that, however. I had to correct the bad performance appraisal. My manager would have none of it. Attempts on my part to rewrite it, softening some of the negative comments, were greeted with derision. To be sure, there were elements of truth to the P.A., but I felt the picture of me that emerged was a cruel caricature. I finally realized that I had no alternative. I had to tell him about Parkinson's. When I brought up the subject, I told him that I had mentioned it to his predecessor, and that he had seemed unconcerned.

"It's getting worse now, as you can see," I said. "Parkinson's is starting to affect my job performance."

"I don't want any phony excuses out of you," he snapped. "Just get down to work and forget about excuses."

I bought a bit of time when I told him about changing doctors, but his reaction was disappointment at not being able to put the blocks to me. I wasn't getting anywhere with him: once his mind was set on a course of action, he would not let facts alter his goal. Unfortunately, he was determined to get my team as well as me.

In fairness to my manager, I must say that I was pretty insufferable at this time. I was by no means a model employee. Despite my efforts not to put my foot in my mouth, or to be too quick with my tongue, I was not totally successful. As I mentioned earlier, our personalities fundamentally clashed. But there was more to it than that. We came from different business cultures. At Wood Gundy and at Molson's, individualism was encouraged and a strong independent personality could flourish. At Molson's there were only three levels between me and the chairman. At the bank there were six. It was extremely hierarchical and there were incredible internal politics. It was a business culture where you stuck to the rule book. My manager had grown up in the bank, loved it, and to an extent had the affection reciprocated. He was a living example of the company man that William H. White had so successfully personified in his 1956 book *The Organization Man,* and he was always trying to ingratiate himself with senior executives. He knew and followed to the letter, the precise rules set down in the bank's *Manual of Routine Procedure.* From his point of view I was a hazard. For example, the bank has financial reporting requirements in virtually all loan agreements and financial tests, such as working capital ratios, tangible net worth, etc. Most bank employees had systems, ranging from simple to complex, that ensured that they could check to see if the reports had arrived on time and if the tests had been met. He asked me one day to describe my "bring forward system," as these things were called.

"It's up here," I said, pointing to my head. And so it was. I kept track of the requirements for my portfolio of companies in my head, without the benefit of hard copy. For him, this was a shocking violation of the system, and pure arrogance on my part to believe that I could keep in my head all the key dates when borrowers had to have their financial reports in.

In this uncongenial environment I was incapable of judging how much of my difficulties came from the job itself, which I hated, and how much came from my Parkinson's. I felt paranoid, always looking over my shoulder and anticipating the future with apprehension, afraid of what the boss was going to do. Neighbours commented that I looked defeated when I left for work in the morning, and I felt it. Coming home in the evening, I looked like the living dead, an automaton. About the only thing that kept me sane was a regimen of exercises that I had started in 1982 to lose weight—I had stopped smoking cigarettes then too.

I thought that things might have been tolerable if this damned Parkinson's wasn't sapping my strength and leaving me without energy as the day wore on. I did not have the energy to fight for a job that would be suited to me. I must have presented the image of a downtrodden clerk in one of Kafka's novels.

In the spring of 1984, I remembered a Scotiabank personnel policy: if an employee believes he has been unfairly dealt with by his manager, he has the right to appeal an adverse performance appraisal all the way up to the chief executive officer of the bank. I was six levels from the top. I knew that although the policy was in place, managers are reluctant to set aside or modify their subordinates' decisions. No one likes to rock the boat.

I prepared my case. I based it on three points:

- bank had not followed through on its commitment to move me over to Corporate Banking, leaving me in Credit, a role in which I was fundamentally unsuited;
- the personality clash with my manager was producing a distorted picture of me in my P.A.;

- Parkinson's disease was a mitigating factor as it was causing both physical and mental changes in me.

My first appeal was to the senior vice-president in charge of the credit function and was unsuccessful, as was my second appeal to the executive vice-president in charge of the division, the man who hired me. (When I encountered him at a Visitor's Day at Camp Gay Venture, Emily's summer camp, he said without a crack of a smile, "I didn't think we paid you enough to send your kid here!") I had thought that my case was a strong one and that its merits would be recognized by probably the first and certainly the second without question. I was shattered when they scoffed and turned me down. The odd thing was, the quality of my work was improving. I had done the entire credit presentations for two large and complex credits that went straight to the chairman of the bank for approval, bypassing the regular process. I was complimented on these reports.

My next step up in the appeal process was to Peter Godsoe, the vice-chairman of the bank. It was three down and three to go. I felt sure I had a strong case, but I wasn't optimistic. He had been a supporter of Esther's in her school board election campaigns, as had many associates at the bank. However, quite rightly, he maintained a Great Wall of China between what went on inside the bank and after-hours socializing.

After I put my case to Godsoe, he smiled and said, "Bill, you're not cut out to be one of the sea-anchors of credit, and Parkinson's is an extra burden on you. I know you have put your case unsuccessfully down the line. Those people report to me. I would have a revolution on my hands if they knew now that you won your appeal. Leave it with me. Wally Meinig will be my point man on this."

I was elated. It was a reprieve. Men and women competed to work for Meinig. I had known him earlier when I was at Molson's where he was senior vice-president in charge of Canadian regions; now at the bank, he was senior vice-president in charge of administration for corporate banking.

Meinig, a sympathetic and realistic man, was an ideal mentor. His daughter had just finished medical school and was interning so he had ready access to expert knowledge of Parkinson's. He also had a real interest in what was happening to me. "Bill, I am shocked by the change in your personality. You have become introverted; what's become of the fun-loving raconteur and bon vivant we all liked so much?"

He was right, I had become introverted. There had been a personality change in me. It was not the first one. As a boy, I had not been outgoing and gregarious. My father had seen to that. The elixir of praise and support was an unknown tonic when I was growing up; the standard medicine doled out by Father was of the awful tasting patent variety hawked by shills as cure-alls—a mixture of ridicule and put-downs mixed with alcohol. I had to work at being extroverted from the time I met Esther. It wasn't fake, but a gradual discovery of my own nature. By the time I was at Molson, it was a natural part of what I had to offer at work and in everyday life.

In 1978 I had been a founding member of the Alderbrandin de Sienne Society, a fine wine club that was really based on good fellowship. I was included because I was fun to be with and a good storyteller. Now, six years later, I had become withdrawn. One friend told me later, "When I agreed to have lunch with you, I didn't know I'd be doing all the talking, and there still would be there were awkward gaps in the conversation."

I had to tell Meinig that my introversion was part Parkinson's and part depression as a result of my unhappiness with the job.

"Parkinson's is nothing to be ashamed of," he said. You didn't get it by doing or not doing anything. What was dumb was using being hungover as the reason for the tremor. Look at the mess that created. Don't worry about the job. You have enough to cope with getting used to Parkinson's."

Esther had been trying since my diagnosis to persuade me to confront Parkinson's, to look it squarely in the face. Wally Meinig said the same thing. "Bill, you have to start telling people who should know that you have

Parkinson's. Don't do it indiscriminately, but tell colleagues and friends."

Over the next few months I took his advice. I had no choice. I had to face the reality of having Parkinson's. The bank now seemed to me to be both Jekyll and Hyde. Meinig was trying to find the best place for me in the organization, while my manager was bound and determined to get me fired or demoted through my P.A. So effectively had my personnel file been contaminated with innuendo that it took several months to place me. Meinig spent countless hours getting a full appreciation of my situation, working every possibility until a place was found.

At the end of the summer of 1984, I went on my annual canoe trip with Howie. As a teenager, I had spent five summers at Camp Stephens on Lake of the Woods, near Kenora, Ontario. The canoe trips were the be best part, and by my last year, I was good enough to go on a two-week trip. I enjoyed being in the wilderness and loved being in a canoe, and having the feeling of being the moving force, with a paddle. In 1980, when I did my first canoe trip with Howie, it had been almost twenty years since my last trip and I was learning by doing it all over again. Howie, who was then 9, had just come back from Camp Voyageur, and was in a very real sense my instructor. For the first time in my life I was conscious of aging. Over the next years we did two trips to Algonquin Park, another to Killarney Park, and a fourth down the Pickerel River. These were in addition to trips we took with Stephen Booth and Tony Graham.

Howie and I always went in the last week of August, because the bugs, black flies, and mosquitoes were sure to be gone, and the lakes and rivers were not crowded with campers. The weather was usually fine: only once in five years did it rain. That was on the first trip. I had read a wilderness book that included some weather forecasting tips. When you see fracto-cumulus clouds, the author assured me, it will not rain. The only problem was that I wrongly identified the clouds. We woke the next morning to pouring rain. There was not far to go, and we made the best of it by discovering that our life jackets were quite effective as "wet suits" in keeping our upper bodies warm. To this day, whenever I make a weather forecast, Howie will say "fracto-cumulus clouds, Dad?"

Over the winter of 1980-81, after our first trip, I had bought a sixteen-foot cedar strip canoe, with clear fibreglass overlaid on the cedar, from Albert Maw of Northland Canoes in Huntsville. I didn't want Esther to think that I was overspending, so I told her that I had won it at the Sportsman's Show. She didn't fall for it, particularly when Albert called to say the canoe I had ordered was ready.

(The canoe has aged more easily and gracefully than I have. Howie still maintains that the canoe is half his.)

It was on these trips that I developed my ideas about decent meals on canoe trips. Why endure freeze-dried foods or Kraft Dinner—which is equally bad—when I could make a vegetable stir-fry and grill a small steak accompanied by a split of decent Burgundy, finishing with a cup of espresso and a good cigar? The joys of cooking bannock over an open fire are highly over-rated, about equal to carrying an unbalanced canoe on a long portage.

Now, as we started the 1984 trip on the Mattawa, I was preoccupied with the implications of Parkinson's and anxious about my future with the bank. I was so distracted by my manager's obsession with finishing me off that I thought it would drive me to a nervous breakdown. Images of his face appeared in my mind for the first day and a half of the trip. Not even my worst encounters with my father had that effect on me.

We put in at a Provincial Park near North Bay and took the sixty miles downriver in three days. Howie did a lot of planning for the trip and was the navigator, and on portages he had to carry the canoe as well. I was starting to stumble a bit, and could no longer manage them safely. In addition, the tremor that was in both sides of my body was a real irritant. There was no point denying or hiding the effect Parkinson's was having on me and for the first time I talked to Howie about it.

Howie was amazingly mature for all his youth. His attitude was very different than on past trips when I was in charge. His takeover was subtle but definite. I think I realized for the first time that my future, at least the future I had planned for myself, was behind me. We chatted for hours about the change Parkinson's was making in the family, particularly in my expectations. The fun and pleasure of the trip was not dampened even when we finished in pouring rain, chilled to the bone and soaking wet. We abandoned our plan to stay in a campsite and checked into a motel where we made inappropriate jokes about refugee families from the third world as we hung our soggy gear about the room to dry, started our gas stove, and cooked a late lunch. The trip was a success for both of us and Howie had developed a real love for canoe-tripping, so much so that his later high school summers were spent as the lead tripper at a girls' camp. But I realized that this was probably going to be my last canoe trip. My stamina was fading, walking was getting more difficult, and I had lost the will.

About the same time, I sold my fifteen-foot Albacore sailing dinghy to Tony Graham, our good friend and cottage neighbour at Blue Sea Lake, for exactly what I had paid for it thirteen summers before. I had never been a successful competitive sailor, but I used to go out sailing every day at Blue Sea with Tony, initially with me skippering. I also used to sail the Albacore single-handed. I was no Joshua Slocum or Francis

Chichester, and sailing alone called for a dexterity and agility that I no longer had. The realization that I wasn't up to demanding physical exercise where decisions I made affected someone else was a let-down. But it was reality, hard reality. The sailing involved a trade-off: if I could not skipper the boat, I could at least have the enjoyment of being the crew. Almost unconsciously, I was beginning to accept the reality of Parkinson's. I was never as good at the tiller as Tony anyhow! (It's amazing how easily that rationalization came.) Selling the sailboat was depressing, but I still sail most days at Blue Sea with Tony at the tiller.

Early in 1985 my father died. We had not grown any closer over the years and I had little affection for him. He was a crude, bigoted man who was always impressed with his own opinions. He was constantly putting down other people for their views, even if his were patently wrong. As he saw himself passed over for promotion time after time, his bitterness grew exponentially, particularly against the men "who were out to get him." It was extreme enough to be called paranoia and had a terrible effect on the family. He drank too much for a long period of time. No, I will not permit the last vestige of filial piety in me let him off that easily. He was an alcoholic and was subject to intense vitriolic rages that left Mother and me shaking with impotent fear.

An incident in 1956 when I was 13 illustrates his penchant for violence. Father had bought a new set of golf clubs. The old set was on his basement workbench, waiting to be discarded, or so I thought.

"How difficult would it be to bend the shaft and break it?", I wondered. It turned out not to be hard at all, once I had put one end in a vise and tightened it. In no time, it snapped in two. Just then, Father appeared at the top of the basement stairs.

"What in Christ's name do you think you are doing?" When I told him, he turned into another person, like Dr. Jekyll and Mr. Hyde. He flew into a rage, the intensity of which I had not seen before or since.

He picked up one of the pieces of the now-broken golf club and chased me around the basement brandishing it like a club. Screams of invective were pouring out of his mouth—he must have been close to foaming. He stopped only after he had drawn blood with the rough metal end of his weapon: a deep four inch gash on the back of my right hand. Mother had been watching this spectacle with helpless tears cascading down her face, screaming "Stop ... stop, both of you!"

"Jimmy, look at what you have done. You have mutilated my son. We'll have to take him to a hospital to get it stitched"

"As usual, Betty, you don't think before you open your mouth. The doctors would ask how it happened."

I still have a prominent scar to remind myself of the event.

Father had always liked big, powerful motorboats. When he was 78 in 1981 he bought a twenty-foot boat with a two-hundred horsepower engine. I told him that someone his age had no business with a boat that big or powerful.

"If I had wanted your opinion, I would have asked for it. You are just like your mother, opening your mouth and talking without thinking if anyone is going to listen."

In 1982, he had a serious stroke. My reaction to the news verged on indifference. He never fully recovered, perhaps because he was "too busy" to take speech and physiotherapy.

The next summer, as he and Mother were leaving the Safeway dock at Kenora, the boat rammed a retaining wall, throwing them both into the water. Mother broke both ankles and wrists, while Father was physically unharmed. Like a small child caught stealing candy in a store, he said to the Ontario Provincial Police officer who investigated the accident: "I opened her right up."

When I went out to Winnipeg to visit them in November, mother's breaks were completely healed and she was caring for Father. She said, "Someone has to look after your father, Bill, he can't look after himself."

Shortly after the accident he began the move to another world, of which he was the only inhabitant. His last two years were spent there.

In some ways, I feel he had it coming to him, after ruining my youth. Yet, even he did not deserve the silent agony that was his destiny.

Father died on January 30, 1985 a day before his eighty-second birthday, in the middle of the night. Mother phoned at six in the morning with a short message: "Bill, your Father is dead." I told her I would get the first plane out to Winnipeg.

When I arrived later that morning, all evidence of Father having lived in the house on Cordova Street for thirty-one years was gone. "Clothes, papers,... What use are they, Bill?" It was tragic that Mother could dispense with the man she had been married to for almost forty-two years with a few garbage bags. She said, "I've got the memories I want. Please don't ask or talk about the kind of father or husband he was."

The funeral, against my wishes, was held in a funeral home. I read a lesson and the congregation sang "Abide with me." Mother had a reception at home after the service. A lot of people came, but the talk was not of him. He was already forgotten.

His death did not have much of an effect on me. It was like closing a book that had gone on too long and finally reached its end. I had no pleasant memories of him, only bitter ones.

Finally, in January 1985, the bank was able to place me in a new department. I was moved to Precious Metals Marketing. My new manager, David Turner, had a broad understanding of neurological conditions because he was an epileptic. He and his boss Larry Mason, a senior vice-president in the investment banking division, made a real effort to accommodate me. My position was a make-work one in the sense that they weren't expecting much from me, and I did not disappoint them in that regard, even though I tried to make a contribution.

But I still had to cope with depression. It is one thing to say that I understood that the cause of my depression was at least partly due to a chemical imbalance in my brain. It is quite another to accept that. There were external factors influencing my depression: the sheer shock of learning that I was imperfect and my former rotten-job attitude being the most important. These factors were not cleared up in the short while after I became aware of them.

Once in my new job, I was left alone for five months to recuperate and regain my mind. I was given permission to do some political work. That was a very unusual step, perhaps implicit recognition on the bank's part that I had been ill-used.

At this time there was impending election for the provincial government. The long-time Progressive

Conservative premier of Ontario, Bill Davis, had just stepped down as leader. I was treasurer of the Progressive Conservative Association for our local riding, St. David, and was deeply involved in the planning of the nomination convention to select a new candidate for the riding. Esther and I had gotten to know Julian Porter through Esther's municipal election campaigns, and she urged him to run for the nomination and offered her support.

I became Julian's eyes and ears on the St. David executive until the end of March when he won the nomination handily. From then until the end of June my time was spent as the chief financial officer of Julian's campaign as the Conservative candidate in St. David in the 1985 provincial election. I began to recharge.

Julian Porter, who combined implausible good looks with a famous ability as a storyteller and speaker, was one of Toronto's leading civil litigation lawyers and had long been one of the Progressive Conservative Party's most promising personalities. Politics ran in the family; his father Dana had been attorney-general in the government of Leslie Frost.

We gave two coffee parties for Julian during the nomination campaign, and Howie got involved as well. Just 14 at the time, he had so much fun that he skipped school on the basis that the campaign was educational. Esther went out canvassing with Julian several times.

Julian, and one or two of the other Porter people, knew that I had Parkinson's, and they were concerned that I not push myself too hard or too long. Each day, I would walk from the bank at King and Bay to Julian's campaign office at Parliament and Winchester, about three miles. I would pick up bills to be paid and contributions received, go back to the bank's offices and do the necessary paperwork. It was fun.

As soon as Porter learned that I had Parkinson's, his first thought was for my future: Was the bank treating me fairly? Had we made adequate provision for the future? How could he help? In that respect, Julian epitomizes what Esther's father meant when he said that we should greet the disadvantaged of the world "not with handouts, but with hands outstretched."

Our association with Julian continued. He was a constant supporter of Esther's in her role as a school trustee and raised money, being very generous himself, to finance her three re-election campaigns.

Julian's campaign had the air of Prince Hal in his famous speech from Shakespeare's Henry V, "Once more unto the breach, dear friends, once more...." In the end Julian lost to his Liberal opponent in an election that saw the Tories go down to a resounding defeat.

Early in the campaign, when the money was not coming in as quickly as we would have liked, Julian said to me after a Sunday evening campaign committee meeting, "Bill, do you know the difference between 'joint liability' and 'joint and several liability'?"

"Of course I do, that is basic to the investment business."

"Just so I am sure you understand, explain it to me!"

"In several liability if you and I together owe one hundred dollars and you go bankrupt, I owe fifty dollars. with joint and several liability, I would owe the full one hundred dollars."

"I'm glad you grasp the concept so clearly, Bill. Under the Election Finance Act, the candidate and the chief financial officer are jointly and severally liable for the campaign debts. My wife [the well-known publisher, Anna Porter] takes a dim view of having to pony up any money at all to cover campaign expenses. I'm sure Esther would be just as upset."

"Upset. Christ, she would be furious."

"Then get out there and get the money in!"

We did get the money in, and after the election was over and lost, Julian and I held a lunch at the Albany Club for the fund-raisers. Altogether, they had raised over $135,000; we thought a thank-you was in order.

It was a convivial group that included Hal Jackman, the godfather of Toryism in Ontario, and Conrad Black, already by 1985 outgrowing his entrepreneurial training wheels. He was now favouring Julian and the other lunchers with his pontifications on sundry subjects including the propriety of full funding for separate schools, an initiative taken in the last days of the Davis government that had contributed to the Tory defeat.

During the drinks before lunch, I was chatting with Douglas Lissaman, now a judge, who said, referring to my tremor, "that must be one hell of a hangover, Bill."

Scarcely believing what I heard myself say, I replied, "That's no hangover Douglas—I have Parkinson's disease." Poor Doug's jaw dropped and for the first time I had known him, he was at a loss for words. If he felt badly, I felt worse. Yet, it was the first time I had admitted to anyone who didn't know me well that I had Parkinson's. There was truly a watershed aspect to my comment. I had come out.

"Coming out" was a complex process that I did not fully understand at the time. By the time of the Porter campaign, Parkinson's was readily apparent to anyone who cared to look. The evidence included a tremor in both hands, limping with both feet, the beginnings of the Parkinsonian mask, and worsening of my handwriting. But I did not consciously decide to "come out," and there wasn't any external social pressure as there is with certain elements of the gay community. My decision was not explicit, nor were there any implicit factors present. It just seemed like a good idea at the time. I think that Esther's constant urging was probably the key factor.

Looking back on the years 1984-85, I see they were for me a time of rebirth and regeneration, much like a caterpillar metamorphosing into a butterfly. Not that I changed into a thing of beauty; quite the contrary. My Parkinsonian mask became more expressionless, my walking became more irregular and my tremor worsened. It was more of an intellectual and spiritual metamorphosis. I didn't judge people quite so quickly and began to seek out compromise and accommodation. The change came about for two reasons. With the death of my father I began to realize the extent of his negative influence on me—particularly his tendency to be judgemental and bigoted in belittling other people. And I had seen both Peter Godsoe and Wally Meinig deal me and my Parkinson's generously and imaginatively, taking risks and placing less weight on the conventional wisdom about me. I tried to learn from them.

CHAPTER FOUR

A Non-practising Intellectual

My next three and a half years working at the bank were spent in relative peace and obscurity in the gold department, developing new products, while my Parkinson's got worse. Since I now had gone public, I no longer had the stress of trying to hide my condition. Nonetheless, I was an enigma to the people at the bank. They did not know what I was or was not capable of doing. And I did not always know what I could do, and I could not tell how people reacted to me. One of the challenges of Parkinson's, as well as many other chronic medical conditions, is the inability of the sufferer to distinguish the rate at which his or her condition is "progressing." Partly this is because, as a patient, you usually don't have a set of objective standards against which to regularly measure or test yourself. But also it is because you really don't want to know. Denial is subtle and pervasive. You say to yourself, "Parkinson's won't progress in me. I'm different." Of course we are all different, but there are immutable laws to which we are all subject. Denial is a reaction to fatalism or determinism.

One of my early assignments was to work out, or collect, on a loan to a gold producer which we were afraid was soon going to become uncollectible. Some years before, the bank had been overeager to increase its loans to junior mining companies, particularly those in Quebec. This was one that had not been successful.

With the assistance of the bank's mining engineer, we analyzed the reserve report, which detailed the size of the ore body, the grade of the ore and the mining plan, showing how and in what order the ore would be mined. On these bases alone, and even with optimistic gold price forecasts, the mine would have had trouble repaying its loan. We traveled to Quebec with the mining engineer, went over the reserve report and mining plan in detail, and inspected the mine.

Scrambling about in a gold mine several thousand feet below the surface was not something that I had looked forward to. But, for the first time I encountered a Parkinsonian truth: Parkinsonians have less difficulty walking on uneven ground or walking up stairs or up a ladder, as compared to level ground. The bank had been concerned about the problems Parkinson's might cause me on this business trip, but none arose.

I had to bring myself up to speed on the whole business of gold loans, exchange for physical, forwards, and a peculiar transaction known in the department as "slow spot." It was a challenge, but after I realized that all these concepts involved the time value of money, it was straightforward.

It was pretty obvious that my managers at the bank were not giving me much to do. The reason, not obvious to me at the time, was, of course, Parkinson's. In a chronic condition like Parkinson's the patient is often the last person to recognize and acknowledge the symptoms. I really didn't know or perceive what was happening to me. I was, to a large degree, unaware of my tremor, limping, facial contortions, and other Parkinson's symptoms. But my bosses were concerned about how the bank's customers would react to someone with this disconcerting appearance. So I was given desk jobs. The principal one was an apparently simple yet complex assignment task: to see if I could come up with some new products for the bank to market. I did develop one product that I thought had considerable appeal. It was a "zero interest gold loan."

In spite of the completed product-development assignment, I was still left with little to do. Instead of just sitting on my thumb, I began to read voraciously. The number of periodicals that the bank subscribed to was almost without number, ranging from The Wall Street Journal and The Economist to arcane newsletters dealing with politics and economics around the world. At home I read books on history, politics, and intellectual history. I did not recognize it at the time, but I was beginning to adapt my life to Parkinson's. As I was constrained in my job by my physical limitations, I was discovering that intellectual activity had no constraints.

How could I put my newly acquired knowledge to good use? One way was to write. I started by writing speeches for Esther to give at the Board of Education. She only used one of them because she said they were too redneck—I considered myself a Burkean Conservative. And, to be honest, I think she resented my interference in her job.

I also began trying to write gold market letters for the bank. Reading them over now, over ten years later, I think they stand up pretty well, but the bank eventually decided against using them because I was unwilling to remove my political bias from the commentary and the bank thought, probably rightly, that right-wing commentary would be poorly received by some of their clients. I tried a couple of other large-scale writing projects for the bank, but ultimately they went nowhere. Looking back, I can see that I was trying to develop a new range of interests, and I can also see that the bank was giving me a tremendous amount of freedom.

I am often wrong, but rarely in doubt. This characteristic, which could be described variously as strong-willed, individualistic, or pigheaded, often has gotten me into trouble but it can also be a great source of strength. It gives me the conviction to be a strong advocate for the argument I am making at the time. But in retrospect, I can see that at this time, at the bank, the stress of having Parkinson's, combined with the psychological effects of the medications I was on, clouded my judgement and allowed me to ignore the merit in the bank's position and perhaps, worse, permitted me to overstate my case. Also, I hadn't yet developed the team-player attitude that is so important in any endeavour, although I had been working for large companies for two decades. I am reminded of Barbra Streisand's response to Mike Wallace on 60 Minutes when he asked her why she had been a patient in analysis for twenty-five years. She replied, "I guess I'm a slow learner.

My intellectual growth at this time was undisciplined, without critical judgement being applied. I was so keen on my newly acquired knowledge and intellectual activity that I was blind and deaf to even to the most constructive criticism. I was the loner, the outsider: in the world, but not of it.

I later discovered that the bank was at its wits end about what to do with me. Now, I can understand their problem. My Parkinsonian symptoms were increasingly obvious: the expressionless mask, limping, tremor, involuntary micro-naps, and indistinct speech. David Turner, my manager, had taken the unusual step of consulting Esther, asking her what I was capable of and what I was not. He told her his frustration at asking me to revise material, only to have me resubmit to him virtually unchanged.

I had been unaware that my symptoms had apparently increased dramatically over that winter. It was some time before I discovered that this was a result of Deprenyl, a new medication that for me had the effect of magnifying the adverse effects of other drugs as well as causing some personality changes. Consequently, at the same time that I was undergoing a good deal of intellectual growth, I was losing my critical judgement.

I had begun taking involuntary micro-naps during the work day—the result, as I later discovered, of medications. One of those quick snoozes was responsible for what could have been a serious car accident in the summer of 1986. Emily and I, together with Sir, (the Airedale terrier who had replaced our first Madam—we would have a second Madam later on), had left for Toronto Blue Sea Lake about 4:30 in the morning on the last Friday in June. Near the town of Hastings I dozed off as we were coming to a stop sign. I ran into, and partly under, a large Beatrice Milk truck. Luckily, no one was hurt. There was a longish delay as we waited for the police, had the car towed to a body shop, and arranged for repairs.

The police chief of Hastings took us to Norwood, about ten kilometres away so we could rent a car and resume our journey. Although there was no rush, he turned the flashing light on as well as the siren and was going at least 140 km/hr. Just as he was telling us that, in thirty years as a policeman, he had "never fired a shot in anger, son," he asked me to put his handcuffs in the glove compartment. As I did so, I could not help noticing that it was full of ammunition. When I pointed out the seeming discrepancy, his laconic reply was a gruff "never hurts to be prepared, son."

The incident frightened Emily so much that she would never drive on the highway with me again. And she had good reason to be frightened: had the micro-nap occurred on a major highway, the accident could have been fatal.

This was an important stage in the progress of Parkinson's in my life. Something had happened as a result of the medication I was taking for Parkinson's, and I had no one to turn to. Still, I did not want the police to notice that I had Parkinson's. My driver's licence might be taken away. The policeman certainly didn't even hint at that, thank heavens!

At about this time a new weekly newsmagazine had started up called Seven Days. A Conservative party friend of mine, Warren Armstrong, had some connection with the promoters of the magazine and knew that they were looking for a columnist on political affairs. He suggested me and the editors took me on sight unseen. The magazine lasted thirteen weeks and I had thirteen articles published. I used the nom de plume Josephine Churchill because the bank, as noted earlier, was not keen on employees publishing articles with a political viewpoint. The topics were as diverse as the Iran-Iraq war, arms control, foreign policy, Canadian politics, and the school system.

I soon settled into a routine for writing the articles. The deadline was noon Thursday. As I was now sleeping no more than five hours a night, I would get up at five a.m. and work on the column until seven. After the first few weeks, the column would be finished by my self-imposed deadline.

This was a positive consequence of my adapting to Parkinson's. My habit of writing in the morning is now firmly entrenched in my daily routine.

One project that captured my imagination was totally unrelated to work of any kind. Starting in 1974, I developed a growing interest in drinking fine wines and cooking wonderful meals. In the winter of 1986-87 after some encouragement by friends, I put together a cookbook, The Great Menu Book, and had hopes of getting it published. Anne Lindsay had been very successful with her books for The Heart and Stroke Foundation. Why, I wondered, couldn't I do the same for either the Movement Disorders Clinic or the Parkinson's Foundation?

The first installment had four menus: a meal we'd had after the trip to Buffalo, a small lunch party, coping with New Year's Day, and Gourmet Cooking on a Canoe Trip. Toronto Life magazine bought the most unlikely menu, the canoe trip one. It was a satirical menu, aimed at the environmental 'deep thinkers' who always had a solution to every problem. It began, "We are Rolls Royce campers and proud of it."

I couldn't get any interest in the project as a fundraiser from the Parkinson Foundation or the Movement Disorder clinic, but I ran off about fifty copies for friends. It was a hit with them and I printed a second installment a few years later.

It's ironic that I would try to put out a cookbook at just the time that I was losing my sense of smell and taste. That happens to most Parkinsonians, but I did not know that. Its one of the cruel things in life—and dangerous too—if you lose the use of those two vital senses. Imagine not being able to tell if bacon is rancid, eggs rotten, or if you have put too much or too little spice in a dish you are cooking.

It was one thing to write about current affairs or even cooking. It was quite another to write on theology. We had been going to Christ Church, Deer Park for almost twenty years. I had been active as a warden, as chair of a committee that recommended a new pipe organ, and as a delegate to Synod, the governing council of the diocese. Now my faith, such as it was, was evolving. It had been an unquestioning one, accepting the traditions and rituals of the Anglican Church in which Esther and I had both grown up, and based on my admiration of individuals who happened to be Christian, a sort of personalized ad hominem argument. The change, and it was a profound one, involved a shift from asking bitterly and selfishly, "Why me, God?" to asking "Why not me, God?"

I was asked to preach a sermon on Reformation Sunday, October 25, 1987, at Christ Church Deer Park, our parish church. The topic was the need for absolute moral standards and the folly of ethical relativism. My peroration...

> We can conclude, or at least I can, that whenever men or regimes start to impose ideas on people, the insidious process of human engineering begins, shoveling flesh and blood around like soil or concrete. Pushing people around seems to be peculiar to socialism, whether of the Russian variety, the German National Socialist kind or the perverse and sinister ethnic socialism in South Africa known as Apartheid. It was set up by the social psychology department of Stellenbosch University. Other types of state socialism in black Africa have usually been legitimized by university intellectuals. So, beware of the intellectual. Far from being non-conformists, they are ultra conformist within the circle whose approval they seek. En masse, this makes them dangerous as it lets them create intellectual climates which can generate irrational and sometimes violent courses of action. Remember that people should come before ideas, not the other way round.

I thought the sermon was successful. However, afterwards when I listened to a tape recording of the sermon, I realized that my voice was becoming a monotone and I was starting to rush words together.

So this was why people would ask me to repeat what I was saying!

My physical appearance was beginning to be disconcerting to others. This was principally dyskinesia, a side effect of my medications, but akinesia (poverty of movement) and (bradykinesia) slowness of movement were also occurring in perverse combination. I did not realize it at the time because I rarely looked in a full-length mirror, and people did not want to hurt my feelings. This all gave rise to an unusual combination: I was going though spiritual and intellectual growth at the same time that I was deteriorating physically. The odd thing was that I was not conscious of this peculiar juxtaposition. This too was a form of denial.

My intellectual transformation was not the only positive thing that happened to me in these years. My friend Stephen Booth had married Gillian Rowan-Legge, whose family owns a share of a salmon fishing camp on the Upsalquitch River, the first New Brunswick tributary of the famous Restigouche River. Stephen invited me to join him on his in-law's fishing party. That first year we drove down in two cars. The party comprised Stephen, Ted and Michael Rowan- Legge, Philip Arthur, David Thornton, and me.

On the first day we drove as far as Rivière du Loup on the south shore of the St. Lawrence. We stayed at the Auberge de la Pointe, with rooms that had a superb view of the St. Lawrence River and the spectacular sunset. In the morning we saw Beluga whales surfacing midway across the river. As it was a Sunday morning, Stephen celebrated Holy Communion before breakfast at 7:15, which gave the day a good start.

Tension mounted as we entered the Matapaedia Valley, through which flows one of Quebec's great salmon rivers to its junction with the fabulous Restigouche. Over lunch at the Restigouche Hotel, the locals were full of optimism. That wasn't very surprising considering that the regional economy is dependent on the sport fishery.

We arrived at the camp at about 3:30p.m., with the temperature in the mid 90s Fahrenheit. We unpacked, assembled our tackle, had pre-dinner drinks, and then ate dinner.

The experience of three and a half days fishing produced some interesting juxtapositions: fishing tackle that was a combination of hi-tech graphite rods and flies that hadn't changed much since the turn of the century; guides who lived apparently contented lives of rural poverty and "sports" who lived sophisticated lives of conspicuous consumption. My juxtaposition was Parkinsonian and physical. I experienced for the first time the excruciating pain of having my toes turn under themselves for periods of time, usually no more than twenty minutes. This was the first dyskinesia, literally "bad movement," I had known. It happened while I was out for a run with the Rowan-Legge brothers. The cure was simple, but had until I got back to civilization. Two capsules of lithium carbonate daily, a medication usually associated with bipolar depression, did the trick.

I also experienced a sense of community. Everyone on our party knew I had Parkinson's, but they made no special efforts to accommodate me, except for helping me get in and out of canoes. I was accepted without reservation. For the first time in years, I felt good about life, and the trips I made to Waquita over the next few years were great occasions to develop and enjoy wonderful friendships and to develop a serious interest in the art of fly fishing.

I killed no salmon that first year, but one rainy evening I had one on for ten minutes before I lost it. A few years later, I wrote a short story called "My Ghillie" in which I used Stephen as the model for an ideal fishing guide.

> On that same first evening, after a camp meal that will never be forgotten, in the pouring rain, we went downriver to the Boyne Pool.
>
> "I would use a number ten Silver Rat, high water version, sir."
>
> Hours passed, casting through rain to no avail. Utterly unlike a New Brunswick guide, he watched every cast, advising and untangling wind knots with just the right mixture of deference, sarcasm

> and respect, surrounding each comment like a caul.
>
> After three hours, even my patience was being stretched. Suddenly my reel started screaming as the salmon that had set the hook in his mouth took of upriver. Dunne poled the canoe to shore, always with an eye on the fish, issuing quick, terse commands:
>
> "...Rod down ... take up the slack ... let him run ... don't let him tie your line around that deadhead .... bring him in, sir ... congratulations sir, you have a twelve pound salmon."

In the spring of 1988, everyone recommended that I start seeing a psychiatrist. Everyone was Esther, Dr. Polak, and David Turner, my manager. Three people may not be "everyone," but to me it seemed as if they were all ganging up on me. The reason was twofold: the depression that I had been experiencing in the past couple of years just would not go away, and I was spending money as if there was going to be no tomorrow. If I kept on spending at the rate I was, my family would soon be impoverished. Over-spending was nothing new to me in 1988—I had little financial self-discipline in my life up to then—but the problem had never been too serious. Now Esther took charge of our finances with a singleness of purpose and dedication that is characteristic. She thought she had me on the straight and narrow in no time.

The idea of going to a shrink was an anathema to me but there was enough pressure on me that I had to go ahead. My first psychiatrist agreed to see me on the basis of a behaviour contract. My side of the bargain was that I would not spend money; his side of the contract was that he would cure my spending and lift my depression. It was an overly simplistic contract, it was oral, and I did not fully understand the implications. Moreover, my psychiatrist and I profoundly misunderstood each other. He habitually smiled and nodded at virtually everything I said, which I assumed indicated approval. Nothing could have been further from the truth. In any event, I had a huge spending spurt, and my psychiatrist fired me. I protested that you don't give someone an umbrella and then take it away as soon as it starts to rain.

The solution to my spending problem was to get rid of my depression. That took two and a half years to accomplish with the next psychiatrist, Dr. Kohl. My sessions with him were much more productive. They focused on looking for the underlying causes of the depression, which were twofold: Parkinson's and my relationship with my now-dead father.

But before that there was a real crisis in the fall of 1988. Esther, having discovered the extent of the recent spending spree, phoned Dr. Lang and said "Get Bill into hospital fast!"

"How soon?" Lang said.

"Yesterday", she said.

My Parkinson's medications had disoriented my mind to the extent that I could not count backward from 10, and I was totally confused. First they got me off Deprenyl. I was in the hospital for two weeks while Dr. Lang and his colleagues, including shrinks from the Western, figured out that Deprenyl was the principal reason for the deepening of my depression and my personality change. That was the simple, and it turned out, correct solution. It provided some short-term relief.

It is now clear to me that the mixture of Deprenyl with the other medications I was taking had produced the chemical imbalance in my brain that had caused the undesirable effects on my behaviour and personality. Another side effect was the magnification of my dyskinesia. It turned out that not enough was yet known about the effects of Deprenyl, indeed about many of the other available psychotropic drugs, on the functioning areas of the brain. This singularity was the first of many I would experience over the next decade. Fortunately, it was the by far the most unpleasant one.

The fundamental problem remained: my Parkinson's symptoms were going through a growth phase—they were getting worse quickly and the basic depression was more deeply embedded in me than I had imagined. Involuntary micro-naps now occurred several times a day without warning and my speech was rushed and monotone. My gait was distinctly irregular and there was the tremor in both hands. Work now was an utter sham. That is, the thought that I was accomplishing anything worthwhile at work was a sham.

Sham notwithstanding, in November I had my annual performance appraisal. I was graded "Fully Satisfactory" and given a salary increase. Who were they kidding? It turned out that they were not even kidding themselves. Peter Godsoe, in a file memo, had said that until further notice I was to be graded at that level and to receive salary increases in line with that rating.

While Godsoe's generous gesture insured that I would not suffer financially as a result of Parkinson's as long as I worked, I sensed that the end was near. I was right. On a bitter January day in 1989, I was told that I would go on short-term disability pending long-term disability in six months time. Knowing it was coming did not soften the blow. The brutal way the telling of the news was given to me was shattering. Just leave. There will be no farewell party for you. Don't linger saying good-byes. Just leave.

In retrospect, it is easy, even obvious to see the reason: they did not know how I would react and they wanted to minimize the possibility of an embarrassing scene. Wisely, I went gentle into that good night.

CHAPTER FIVE

Coping With Retirement

In the winter of 1989 I left work with a long-term disability pension. In effect, this meant retiring twenty years early on 60 percent of my then salary of $55,000. The monetary loss would have been shattering if Esther had not had the income from her position as a public school trustee. I had already been feeling guilty because simply by having Parkinson's I had limited our family's economic potential. Promotion had effectively been cut off. Now, our position was retarded even more. Cutting back would be tough, especially with Howard going away to university in a year.

There was another, no less pressing problem. What would I do with my time? There was now all day, every day to fill.

One of the first things I did was to drink. There I was at home all day alone, with spirits always available and an eight-hundred bottle wine cellar in the basement. I didn't set out to get drunk—it was all quite civilized. A drink before lunch. Some wine with lunch; soon it became a bottle—no one need know. Add that to the usual pre-dinner drink with Esther—as a rule I would be sobered up by dinner time—and I was a walking time bomb. And having had an alcoholic father, it would have been all too easy to blame it on him.

I was saved from this disaster by Parkinson's itself. It slowly dawned on me that my speech was worse and my movements much more constrained when I was drinking. At first, in my haze, I put it off to not taking my pills on time. I gradually realized that alcohol was the cause; it was lessening the effectiveness of my drug therapy. I had a decision to make: booze or coping with Parkinson's? I opted for coping with Parkinson's.

In a way, Parkinson's was my ally: one of the things that tends to go with Parkinson's is a less acute sense of smell, and about three-quarters of what we perceive as taste is really smell. Since I could no longer really enjoy all the subtleties and nuances of fine wines, it wasn't so hard to say, "To hell with it, I just won't drink alone any more!"

I didn't stop drinking. I was able to cut back to moderation without difficulty, although if I had carried on drinking heavily much longer it might not have been so easy.

One thing that kept me busy over the next couple of years was looking after family affairs, in particular my father's family. My father had two brothers, Archibald and Harold, and two sisters, Jean who had died some years before, and Louise, who was unmarried and lived not far from us in Toronto. Archibald, the eldest, was by far the most successful member of the family. He had spent his career in the bank of Montreal's Investment Department working in New York and Montreal. He had done well personally in the stock market before being wiped out in 1929, and then rebuilt his fortune. He had married twice, but had no children. His first wife, who had died while riding a camel in Egypt in 1950, was a great-aunt of Esther's. His second marriage was to Helen Edward. In 1975, Arch had been diagnosed with cancer. He said to Helen, "Now, I don't want the family coming down to Montreal and trying to suck up to me on my deathbed. But I do want Bill to come and see me. I have a special job for him."

I arrived in Montreal and went to Arch's house on Rosemount Avenue in Westmount. Aunt Helen took me to his room at once, saying, "He's been looking forward to your visit for days, Bill."

"Bill," Arch said as I entered his room, "as I lie here, I want to tell you that I have decided that you shall be the head of the family after I die. Your responsibilities include looking after Louise's finances. I am giving you a sealed metal box. It is yours. Take it to Louise. She will tell you more. In the meantime, I want to give you the bloodstone seal ring AT [for Archibald Thomas]—my grandfather and his father—gave me."

The scene was bizarre, like something out of The Godfather. The box was about the size that would hold a forty-ounce bottle of whisky, and it was heavy. It was bound up with twine, each intersection being marked with blobs of red sealing wax, jammed down by the impression made by the bloodstone seal. Fortunately, those were still the days before you had to be inspected by a metal detector before boarding an airplane. I got the box back to Toronto and went directly to Aunt Louise. She immediately called her brother to say that the metal box had arrived safely with the seals unbroken.

She then broke the seals and opened the box. There were boxes within boxes, containing coins—there must have been a thousand of them of all shapes, sizes, and descriptions. Some were gold. Louise explained that they were the property of the family and had formed part of the immense collection of William Boyne, a great-uncle of Louise and her brothers and sisters. They had been passed down from grandfather to Arch and now to me. The principle behind the little hoard was that it was a highly mobile reserve fund to be used only if urgently required by the family. Arch had designated me as the next owner and custodian. Louise wanted to keep them in her possession until she died.

I thought nothing more about them for sixteen years, except when Louise would bring them out to show me, which was usually before her brother, my uncle Harold, was making a visit to Toronto. "He's so interested in coins, Bill," she would say with sisterly affection.

Our family was very close to her. In the spring of 1989, shortly after I left the bank, we realized that Louise could no longer look after herself. She was now 92 and had been living in the same upper duplex in North Toronto, three blocks from us, for fifty years. She had been living on her own with some nursing care but the care had broken down, she now was confused, her nursing attendant had not bathed her, the apartment was a mess and she had a weak back. The previous summer, Louise had been quite sick as a result of the heat, and had become mentally unbalanced, thinking she was Grand Duchess Anastasia Romanov, the lost heiress to the Russian throne. Her first words on seeing me when we got back from Blue Sea Lake had been, "Bill, you have a sacred duty to kill Rasputin. Did you hear that knock? It is one of my imperial messengers."

There was some background to this fantasy. Some fifty years earlier, in the late 1930s, Louise and her mother had read everything they could get their hands on dealing with the Russian royal family. During the following five days I heard the same story each evening, with only insignificant variations.

Aunt Louise was loved by all of us, particularly Emily. We hated putting her in a nursing home, but it was the only thing to do. It was left to us to empty her apartment, a task that we put off for a few months because Louise wanted to keep the apartment.

The task was larger than we imagined. Esther and I had never thought of Louise as having much in the way of possessions. How wrong we were. First came the junk—a lifetime's supply of styrofoam trays of various sizes and shopping bags from supermarkets, all arranged by size and store. Then came bottles, bags and other containers, some full, the majority empty. These were the legacies of her everyday life.

Her other life was a fantasy life comprising memories, real and imagined, from her childhood. They were mainly family memories, hagiographical in nature, of her three sisters, four brothers, my grandparents, and other relatives. These and the rest of her things were her spiritual legacy.

In the end, emptying the apartment took two weeks and took much out of us, both physically and mentally. What wasn't there was almost as interesting as what was. Some of her treasures were valueless—twelve bolts of antique silk were ruined by mildew in the basement, fine China and crystal were uniformly chipped where they had come in contact with the spout of the faucet. There were some real treasures, principally associated with two ancestors, Joseph Walker and William Boyne.

Walker, my father's maternal great-grandfather, was a major-general in the Royal Marines, having served under Nelson at Trafalgar and Copenhagen, and later in India. From Walker, Louise had a beautiful Indian mahogany campaign desk inlaid with ivory, two Czech painted-green glass vases and a good deal of family portraiture.

Boyne, whose metal box of coins I had brought to Aunt Louise, was the greatest numismatist in Europe in the nineteenth century. He had lived in England, and then for the latter part of his life in Nice and Florence. The Boyne legacy comprised almost one thousand lithographs and engravings and his entire literary remains, both holographs and printed editions of his numismatic and bibliographical works.

I had seen the prints before. They had figured prominently in Louise's hagiography of the family. Boyne was reverentially referred to as Uncle William even though he died four years before she had been born. The prints were representations of friends of Uncle William, Louise said, although in most cases the subjects, the painter, the engraver, or all three had died long before Boyne was born.

The very best of the art work—two complete sets of engravings by John Martin, Illustrations to Paradise Lost and Illustrations to the Bible—we donated to the National Gallery of Canada. The rest of the prints and all the books were donated to the Thomas Fisher Rare Book Library at the University of Toronto.

Every family has a black sheep. In ours, he was more like a rogue elephant. He was my father's middle brother, Harold. Like his brothers, Harold started off working in a bank, but left to join the federal public service, working in the Department of Veterans Affairs.

He seems to have made a specialty of working in northern Ontario.

He was a pack rat, acquiring collections of many things, but most notably a fine collection of early Inuit carvings, and an extensive collection of firearms and swords. How he acquired and paid for these many things is not known, although it is known that he was bailed out by his brother Arch on many occasions.

In 1948 he was dismissed from his job, dare I say sinecure, for no reason other than "they" were out to get him. The "they" were influential, because the efforts of his brothers James and Archibald to obtain redress went just about as high as one could go in those days. In these years of government restraint, it is difficult to appreciate the prodigious achievement of being fired by the government in 1948.

Harold was a womanizer. That does not render him unique; what is close to unique is the detailed daily record he kept of his dalliances with lady friends and his activity with them before and during his marriage to Winifred and after her death. I point this out not out of any puritan disapproval, but to note that his public service salary, and later, pension could not have kept him in the style to which he had become accustomed.

His avocations were very expensive: collecting and women. At the time of his death in 1989, he had leased warehouse space the size of a five-car garage, and it was jammed full. One of the items stored—and it was an item for which we never found an explanation—was a coffin containing the remains of a Caucasian female. As for women, alive that is, his paramour at the time he died was pregnant and Harold was in the process of establishing a trust for her issue. Only when the baby was born and was black, which neither Harold nor the mother were, was the family able to stop the process.

A discovery that Harold's granddaughter made almost unhinged her. She had asked her grandfather for financial help in going to university, and he had refused. By dint of hard work and sacrifice she was able to go anyway, and one of her fellow students, a young woman with whom she became friendly, was telling her that her tuition and residence fees were being paid by an older man, "old enough to be your grandfather."

It was her grandfather.

Harold's life seemed to be a chain of ignoring his family in crisis while providing for strangers. I would not be telling this story unless there was probable cause to believe that I had been violated by this man and that he took advantage of his sister Louise's good nature. He plundered the majority of our family inheritance.

In July 1991 Aunt Helen, Uncle Arch's widow, died, and in October Aunt Louise died. Louise had specified in her will that the funeral and associated arrangements were to be simple. The unctuous, Uriah

Heep-like individual from the funeral home did not seem to know what I meant by simple. Compounding matters, he thought I needed consolation because of my tremor and speech. When I told him that it was Parkinson's, not grief, that was responsible, he said, "Well, sir we all have our minor Calvaries, our little crosses to bear." Evelyn Waugh was right to satirize the funeral industry in The Loved One. Recently one of north Toronto's community newspapers ran a story on a funeral director whose hobby was being a clown. A perfect example of life imitating art.

Just how interested Uncle Harold had been in the box of coins that I left in Louise's care I was to find out after her death. By then, the coins that in 1975 filled the largish metal box would now not fill a one-pound chocolate box. Harold's son had hinted at the diminution of the coins when, after his father died in 1989, he observed that Harold had sold a number of quite valuable coins over the years.

Apparently, Harold had been looking at the coins on several evenings with Louise, and when she was tired and went to bed, Harold would say: "Ouisee, you just go to bed. I'll put these away." And put them away he did, in his pocket.

I had assumed that something along these lines had occurred, but not on such a grand scale.

I knew that because of William Boyne's reputation, the provenance of the coins would add to their value. I wanted to have the remaining collection valued and went with the small number of the coins—all the gold coins had vanished—that remained to Christie's, the international auction house, when their numismatic specialist was in Toronto in 1993. His first reaction was, "Mr. Harshaw, you are treating those coins very casually. If genuine, they are worth a good deal of money. They are very rare, and in good condition."

He picked up each coin in turn, and when he had examined all nineteen of the Greek coins, he said, "These are all British Museum study reproductions.[4] Had they been genuine, this lot would have been worth over two million dollars. You know, the last time we saw the real things was when we auctioned them for a shady character in San Diego in the late 70s."

My uncle probably thought he was entitled to the money, as he believed he had been dealt with unfairly in several family wills. In fact, he had contested the wills of both his father and his mother on the grounds that the money left to care for his sister Jane, who was schizophrenic and was institutionalized for much of her life, was excessive.

How did I feel when I realized the extent of Harold's scam? Violated. A trust had been abused. How had Harold felt about this? My guess is that the word "guilt" was not part of his vocabulary. He was just one of those people who are amoral and unscrupulous.

My mother was a good friend to us and a loving Granny to our children after Father died. Her remaining years were fun-filled and she showed her sense of humour. The last thirty years with Father must have been like being in a prison without walls. A few years before Father died, Mom had said, "I don't know what has happened to your father. When we were courting, and in the early years, he was so much fun and had a good sense of humour." I think she found it easier to accept Father's point of view rather than provoke an argument that would only be unpleasant.

Esther was becoming increasingly concerned about Mom's health. One day in January 1992 she phoned Mom's doctor to express her concern. This was the only time either of us had interfered in Mom's business. She was shocked when the doctor suggested that Mom had a drinking problem, as her hand trembled. Esther said "Read her chart. You will see that she has Parkinson's!" Esther was shocked that the doctor was not aware of this. On that same day, Mom had a heart attack and died while putting on her coat to go to an appointment with her doctor.

Despite the fact that both Mom and I had Parkinson's, we never had any significant conversation about it. And at that time, only a few years ago, medical science was saying that Parkinson's was not a hereditary condition, although I had evidence in my own family, since my mother's mother also had the condition. Recent research is showing that genetics does indeed play a part in Parkinson's.

Mom's funeral was a proper one, held in her parish church. I read a lesson from Revelation.

At a small reception after the funeral, someone said to me: "how does it feel to be an orphan?"

I responded with a defiant "I'm not an orphan. I am the head of a dynasty." It was not a kind thing to say, but I believe that was a turning point in my life. I finally was on my own.

Back in 1989, when I took my great-great-uncle William Boyne's literary remains over from Louise, the books that most intrigued me were his travel journals. I have not traveled extensively and so his journeys seemed all the more romantic to me. They cover three distinct trips: France, Italy, and Egypt (1845-46); Spain and Portugal (1847); and South Africa (1852-55). Over a year I transcribed all the travel journals, some 50,000 words, and did considerable research on one of Boyne's avocations—the study of Gothic cathedrals. I wound up writing an editorial introduction to the journals and a specific introduction to my great unfinished project: recreating the three weeks Boyne spent with his sister Jane, my great-grandmother, in Rome in November 1845. In working on this material I was able to get a better grasp of the man my older relatives had spoken of in such hushed and respectful terms. He turned out to be a disappointment as a personality, with opinions that would make him a laughing stock today. He was a self-made man, reactionary in politics, condescending to servants, and contemptuous of all those whose station in life was below what he perceived his to be.

The work I did on Boyne and Victorian England was part of my liberation from the bonds of Parkinson's. It's not that my symptoms were becoming any less severe, or that my medications were managing them any better. Indeed, the physical side of Parkinson's was steadily progressing. But I was beginning to use my mind as I had never used it before. I devoured books on history and philosophy in an attempt to understand Boyne and his time. I began to gain an understanding of myself. Even so, it was an unfocused understanding because there was no project that used this insight.

Then, in May of 1990, I went with Stephen Booth to the Toronto Diocesan Synod, which was held at Trent University, just outside Peterborough. Synod is, in effect, the legislature of an Anglican diocese, comprising all the active clergy and lay representatives. I was glad to be part of this gathering even though many of the sessions were admittedly very boring. Stephen spent much of the time tying flies. One evening, when I was ambling back to my room to have a drink with Stephen, I heard Art Brown, a suffragan bishop, like a voice in the wilderness, crying out, "Does anyone have some Scotch?" Good soldiers that we were, we answered "yes," and were invited to bring it along.

That one word changed my life. In the room with Art were Taylor Price, Doug Blackwell, all three of them bishops, and a varied assortment of lay and clerical delegates. These 'evenings of fellowship' as the devotees call them, lasted well into the small hours of the next day, During the night, many stories were told, many true, some apocryphal, and some simply because the teller of the tale thought it was good idea at the time. The best stories were about Esther's father, my late father-in-law, Archbishop Howard Clark. There was warmth and affection, love and respect. I had heard, but not fully realized in what high regard Clark had been held by the clergy, what a positive influence he had been in so many people's lives, and how he was seen as a role model. At the end of the evening, Art said, "Bill, you're not doing anything now. Why don't you write Howard's biography?"

"You can't be serious, Art!"

"I'm very serious, Bill. You're qualified to do it, and you're at loose ends now."

"Loose ends" was a charitable way of describing my life at that point. I was killing time and feeling a bit sorry for myself as Parkinson's continued its conquest of my body. I was beginning to feel that Parkinson's was running my life more than I was.

I needed something to do, a challenging project that would take my mind off myself and direct it to something worthwhile. The idea of a biography seemed ideal. Clark was now an icon of the Anglican Church.

Four decades after he left Ottawa, where he had been Dean of the Cathedral, he was still known as the "great Dean." The years when he had been Primate, that is head, of the Anglican Church in Canada, had been a watershed for the church, and he had an international reputation as an ecclesiastical diplomat, and had been loved wherever he went. He had, moreover, had to deal with challenging medical problems. He had contracted ankylosing spondylitis in his mid-thirties. This is an inflammation of the vertebrae, which is extremely painful. It resulted in his having to be immobilized for nine months while his back and neck fused in 1943-44, when he was 40. As I struggled with Parkinson's I had become interested in knowing how he had coped with a chronic degenerative medical condition. Here was my opportunity.

The only problem was that I had no experience in writing a book, to say nothing of a biography. I did not let that stop me. Objections were brushed aside and on I went. Not everyone was impressed with the idea. The cruelest comment came from one of Esther's cousins. When I told him of my project, he said: "Oh, I guess they couldn't get anyone else to do it."

Who would publish my biography? The Anglican Book Centre ("ABC"), which rather grandly styles itself as "publisher to The Church," seemed the obvious choice, but their initial reaction was anything but enthusiastic.

My first meeting with ABC was held at the home of James Mainprize, the company's editorial director. (The house, by coincidence, had been owned in the 1940s by an aunt of my mother's and was the site of my parents' wedding reception.) Mainprize was cautiously optimistic, but pointed out that clerical biographies, "even of one as distinguished and well-known as your father-in-law" would have a pretty small market. What I did not realize at the time was that Mainprize was the sole professional editor at ABC. His time was at a premium because he had to attend to ABC's line of spiritual self-help books, which were their bread and butter, as well as to their trade books.

I was contracted to produce a manuscript by September 1991. The next problem was how to pay for the research costs. They would be substantial, principally for travel from one coast of Canada to the other. I applied to the Canada Council and the Social Sciences and Humanities Research Council to no avail; I had no Ph.D. and no experience. Then, the Anglican Foundation of Canada came to the rescue with a five thousand dollar grant. I realized how fortunate I was as a first-time author to receive a grant.

My work on the Clark biography involved interviewing a great many people. I had to face the fact that my Parkinson's symptoms, or the side effects of the medications, had a disconcerting effect on many of the people I met who did not know me. It was the same problem I had had at the bank but now more so since many of my Parkinson's symptoms have progressed. My speech was becoming more slurred and indistinct, my handwriting was becoming illegible and dyskinesia was becoming a major problem, taking up a radius of two and a half feet. It occurred mainly when my medications were "on." Most of the time, I would not be aware of the dyskinesia. I wondered why people were giving me such a wide berth on the streets, or indeed, crossed over to the other side of the street to avoid me. I realize now how frightening I must have looked to some people with no knowledge of Parkinson's or other chronic neurological diseases. I would be looked upon as being drunk or on drugs; in any event, a disconcerting sight.

It took me some time until to deal with these problems directly. In retrospect, I don't know why it took me so long to get my act in order. Mostly it was my own apprehension about people's reaction. My solution didn't make the problems go away but did allow me to have something like reasonable encounters with new people. It was a simple matter of saying, "I have Parkinson's. Please excuse my indistinct speech and unusual body movements. I am recording this interview because I cannot write legibly."

I found that people are uneasy with the unknown. When they knew the reason for my peculiar physical behaviour, the people I interviewed were more than accepting, they were accommodating. Nonetheless, many people still did not know what to make of me. When I sent early drafts of chapters or sections to experts for comment, they would almost invariably say "very good" or "looks alright to me." Then, sub rosa they would say to my editor at the Anglican Book Centre that there were problems with the text. Occasionally, they would tell Esther on the understanding that she would not tell me. Quite apart from a lack of intellectual honesty—in fact, downright lying—comments from an unattributed source are worse than useless. As a result I had great difficulty getting honest constructive criticism.

I had thrown myself into the project with single-minded energy—it felt so wonderful to have something worthwhile to do. I turned in a complete draft to ABC in April, fully six months ahead of schedule. At no time did I receive any editorial direction or guidance, either before or after delivering the manuscript. Mainprize had fallen into the same trap that others had: he did not know how to deal with me. When I did not hear from him for two months, I took the unusual step of, in effect, becoming my own editor. I sent out draft chapters, and in two cases the whole book, to experts in the fields the chapters dealt with. By November, 1991 I had a complete new draft of the book ready, and submitted it.

The Rt. Rev. Barry Valentine, Clark's successor as Bishop of Rupert's Land, was an excellent interview subject, a stern critic of various drafts and very concerned as a pastor for my health as I wrote the book and readied it for its eventual publication. He alone of my "editorial readers" separated me as biographer from me as a Parkinsonian and tried to deal with the two aspects separately even while recognizing that the two were parts of the larger whole that was me. As a result of Barry's efforts, the book was much better and we have become friends.

One of the chapters in my original draft had the rather grand (or so I then thought) title "The Provenance of Contemporary Theology." I sent it to Dr. Eugene Fairweather, one of the most distinguished of Anglican theologians, now retired, and followed up with a visit to him at his home in Hortonville, just outside Wolfeville, Nova Scotia.

Eugene had begun his career as a theological enfant terrible in the 1940s. He spent close to half a century based at Trinity College in Toronto as tutor, professor, and later Dean of Divinity, had held a variety of visiting professorships and published enormously, was a leading figure in the ecumenical movement, and had been an observer at the famous Vatican II council of 1965. He was now the grand old man of Anglican theology in Canada.

Dr. Fairweather greeted me on the lawn of his two hundred year-old frame house overlooking the mud flats of the Gaspereaux River. He was quick to point out that "Hortonville is really the original town, so Wolfeville is its suburb rather than the other way around." I absorbed this statement of local historic snobbery in the spirit of humorous irony in which it was delivered. Dr. Fairweather went on to point out that his forebears were Planter stock, a group of immigrants—today they would be called refugees—who antedated the Loyalists' arrival on the scene. The latter group, he said, were arrivistes.

His appearance was quite unlike what I had expected of the doyen of Anglican theology. He looked almost every bit the farmer he was not. His shoes, shirt, and trousers were totally suited to the rural ambience of Hortonville. What gave him away was the silver-grey hair that cascaded over his shoulders and the stylish blue-rimmed eyeglasses. No farmer would be caught alive in that peculiar mixture of styles that suggested a character in a novel. In fact, Fairweather is widely thought to be the basis of the Rev. Simon Darcourt in The Rebel Angels, the first novel in Robertson Davies' Cornish trilogy.

Going into his house through the kitchen, Fairweather pointed out the three honours that meant most to him. They hung over the kitchen sink and were: an honourary doctorate from the Jesuit Regis College, and two letters—one from Pope John XXIII and the other from Archbishop Runcie, then Archbishop of Canterbury, commending him for his work on Anglican-Roman dialogue.

Making our way through books—it seemed that there were so many that the house would collapse without them—we then went into a large glassed-in sun-porch on the second floor. There he had no difficulty persuading me not only that the title of my chapter,

"The Provenance of Contemporary Theology" was incredibly pompous, it was also misleading, and anyway, such a chapter had no business in a popular biography. So out it came. In addition, he spent seven hours pointing out, in the most gracious way possible, errors of fact and interpretation, both subtle and egregious, in the draft of the Clark biography I had sent him. It was an experience to treasure, for Fairweather had a truly encyclopedic knowledge of the subject.

Other readers were similarly generous of their time. Yet not a word came from the Anglican Book Centre until they sent a letter, which I opened on my return to Toronto from my mother's funeral. It informed me that the ABC was unilaterally canceling the contract with me because of the small market for episcopal biographies and the substantial amount of editorial work that my book required. I was shattered. I considered legal action, but then realized that ABC had used the publisher's standard "out" clause in the contract.

Looking back, I now realize that I should have seen it coming. I also realize that the reason the experience was so depressing was that, despite the co-operation I had from Eugene Fairweather and others, I felt alone and without any support for the project itself. Here I was, writing away on a vastly complex intellectual project completely on my own, with no assistance from my publisher who had now rejected me.

I considered giving up the idea of finishing the biography and in fact put it aside for several months. I was feeling pretty low but I slowly realized that, after 117 interviews and much thought, I had found out one of the keys to Clark's success in dealing with his chronic medical condition: set your goals and objectives without regard for your condition and God will let you know if they are realistic. It is a simple faith, but it is not simplistic. Clark had reduced the essentials of his faith to an absolute minimum. Similarly, his goals were not complex. In effect he asked himself how his physical constraint might be an advantage. How did he put that to use? By deciding to spend more time with his children and to strengthen himself intellectually by reading widely in theology and philosophy. He was successful in each of these.

Applying the same principles to myself, my goals became: to get the book published and to find ways to make the most of my physical constraints were an advantage. I had already found one way to accomplish the latter: using my "off" time, when my medication was ineffective and I was more or less unable to move, to read and think.

First I put the biography away for five months in order to gain perspective. Then I asked Archbishop Ted Scott, who had been Clark's successor as Primate and was now retired, to serve as my mentor. This was, for me, an rather unlikely choice, because his political views were at the opposite end of the spectrum from my strongly conservative ones. Scott is known the world over for his advocacy on behalf of the disadvantaged and the oppressed. It was a political and social position that often put him at odds with a good many influential members of the church.

Over the next twenty-one months, Ted's advice and counsel was invaluable to me. He would not let me give up, either in fighting Parkinson's or finishing the book and getting it published. Ted's comments on my manuscript gave me a fresh perspective on Archbishop Clark and his contribution to the life of the church. Ted's support was invaluable to me and to Esther in that difficult time. He first said that I had a responsibility to my late father-in-law, to the men and women I had interviewed, the Church, and to myself to see it through. As well, it was clear that this would be the only biography of Clark that would be written. Ted's support and encouragement gave me the resolve to finish the book. I knew it would not be easy, but now I was determined to succeed.

CHAPTER SIX

Shall We Dance?

From the fall of 1991 onwards, I had the feeling life was closing in on me. I was I suppose, close to paranoia. There was no doubt my Parkinson's was getting worse, particularly akinesia—extreme poverty of movement—and its opposite, dyskinesia—the involuntary shaking that is characteristic of Parkinsonians. Generally akinesia came when my meds went "off." Dyskinesia was a side effect of my meds when they were "on."

Because of akinesia, I was becoming increasingly constrained, as my legs would freeze and immobilize me. My stride would shrink from a normal couple of feet to a few inches and I began freezing in my tracks. This was frightening because it seemed to happen at random, regardless of whether or not I had taken my medications on time.

My ventures out from the house became less frequent and for shorter distances—I would have to estimate the duration of a medson period and guide myself accordingly. I wouldn't dare take the subway during rush hour. And driving was increasingly problematic! After the accident on the way to Blue Sea in the summer of 1988, Emily would not drive with me on the highway, nor would Esther. My physical world was getting smaller.

The attacks of akinesia were not only disconcerting to others; they were also inconvenient, as I was becoming more and more unreliable. It was a struggle to come to terms with this, but the Clark method helped here too. Eventually I realized that the world would not stop if I was half an hour late. I would just get myself to a place where I could sit down and have a cup of coffee and wait until I could walk again. That was like a revelation to me. Yet, it should have been so obvious. Ted Scott said to me that what I should be doing was permitting the world to accept me as I am, not as someone with a barrier around them. "People will accept your disability."

That was all very well. But I did not relish the thought of ending up like the British physicist Stephen Hawking who has the full use of his brain, but who is utterly constrained physically by Lou Gehrig's disease.

The dyskinesia was a side effect of the L-dopa medications Sinemet and Prolapa. The shaking came from involuntary muscle movements in the arms, legs, hands, feet, head, face, and neck. The movements, more like contortions, meant that I needed a clear five feet to walk because the radius of my contorted movement was two-and-a-half feet.

At about this time a friend of mine, the photographer Pete Paterson, took a series of photographs that give, as clearly as pictures can, an indication of the extent of difficulty I had moving about when my meds were off and just how bad dyskinesia was.

In mid-November 1991 Dr. Lang had switched me from regular Sinemet to Sinemet CR, a controlled release form of the medication. Instead of releasing all the L-dopa at once, the CR version released the medication slowly into the bloodstream and then to the brain. It did do that. But it became apparent that I needed approximately 40 percent more of the CR medication than of the regular Sinemet. By now I realized that life was a series of trade-offs. The trade-off this time was more and worse dyskinesia.

The autumn of 1991 was time for another re-election campaign for Esther as school trustee. I wanted to use my newly developed skills as a writer. I worked hard writing speeches, draft after draft, trying to get just the right tone, style, and content. But Esther had her own ideas and was very hard to please. She even wanted to write her own material! I thought it was preposterous! After all, she was only the candidate.

Instead, since workers were scarce that year, I wound up delivering coffee party invitations, putting lawn signs in—and taking them out after the election. Some of our traditional workers committed themselves in other wards, feeling that Esther was not running as hard as she had been in the past. She didn't seem to have the energy to campaign for a sustained period of time, and couldn't go for more than an hour or two without having to take a break. I thought she was getting lazy. What's more, she did not seem interested in the outcome. Esther's financial supporters, however, remained constant. Her fundraisers put in a tremendous effort through all four campaigns to ensure that Esther could finance re-election. This was particularly important by 1991 as I was on my long-term disability pension and so had a substantially reduced income. Allan Portis, a colleague from the bank, joined the campaign as chief financial officer, looking after the financial control and audit functions, and did a super job.

Esther was pessimistic and held her campaign thank-you party before the election. Her voters came through, however, and she was elected to a fourth term as school trustee with a record plurality. Yet, somehow her victory seemed hollow to her. There was little of the enthusiasm, boundless energy, and bounce that had characterized her earlier victories.

I blamed it on the psychiatrist who had been seeing Esther three times a week as a patient in analysis since 1984. She had begun seeing him to help her resolve some problems mainly relating to coming terms with her father's death and with the diagnosis and consequences of my Parkinson's. But now, she would often go for several sessions without a word of feedback from him. In fact, at about this time, Esther was undergoing her own severe depression, which he failed to recognize.

Analysis was not the right sort of therapy for Esther. She concealed very adroitly her main reason for needing help: a fear, verging on paranoia, that she was going mad. She felt that the world was closing in on her, yet there was nothing she knew that was wrong with her. At times, she could not move in crowds or walk up onto a stage. In addition, there were other disturbing symptoms that she tried as much as possible to conceal or disregard. Her energy level was much lower and she could no longer walk for more than a few hundred yards without feeling fatigued. Sometimes she had difficulty walking and maintaining her balance and her eyes were doing strange things—blacking out for short periods of time without warning, for example—and her vision generally was deteriorating.

She was, indeed still is, a superb actress. When the occasion demanded, or at least when she was "on parade," Esther could put on a marvelous performance, stretching her resources to the limit. These virtuoso performances fooled just about everyone, including me and the children.

Her symptoms had first begun appearing about ten years earlier, and Esther had been hospitalized twice to try to get a diagnosis. The second time was in 1984, for a drooping of one side of her face and weakness on her left side. When that cleared up on its own accord, no diagnosis was made. After discharging her from hospital, Dr. Macdonald, the same neurologist who had diagnosed my Parkinson's, said to Esther, "Not much that I can find wrong with you now. Maybe in ten or twenty years you'll turn out having something like multiple sclerosis. Maybe not." Nothing more was said. But seven years later the problems were still there. She had given up on an exercise programme because she simply could not raise either leg. Worse than that, she fell frequently. I later discovered that she would often have to crawl up or down stairs, when no one was watching, because she was afraid of falling down—she could not see to put one foot in front of the other.

In October 1992, Esther had another appointment with Dr. Macdonald and was waiting for the results of some tests. She had heard nothing and was feeling frustrated and anxious.

I said to her, "It's been a week since you saw him. Why don't you telephone him?"

I listened to the call.

"May I please speak to Dr. Macdonald?... It's Esther Harshaw.... Good afternoon, Doctor.... Do you have the results of my test yet?... Yes ... what does that mean?... no doubt in your mind. Thank you. Good-bye."

Tears were streaming down Esther's face. She began sobbing. I crossed the kitchen and hugged her.

"What did he say?"

"Dr. Macdonald said I have demyelinating multiple sclerosis, just as he thought seven years ago."

"Seven years ago! Christ, why didn't he tell you then?"

"Don't get mad at me, Bill. I'm only telling you what he told me."

It was eerie, weird. The same doctor, Ronald Macdonald, was now giving Esther the same sort of bad news he had given me, but this time over the phone. At least she now knew what was wrong with her.

"Do you remember how keen he was about your diagnosis?"

"How could I forget?"

"His voice on the phone just now was enthusiastic!"

To Esther, MS was associated with her namesake aunt, her mother's twin. The aunt's struggle with MS had been a bitter one. Consequently, Esther had blocked that possibility from her mind. Perhaps too she felt unable to cope with each of us having a chronic neurological condition. "Look at the broken towel racks in the bathroom," Esther had said, blaming me for the damage. Only after she had the diagnosis did she confess that she was responsible. Looking back, it is easy to see that the problems she had been having, the deteriorating eyesight, the awkward gait and poor balance, the lack of energy, were all classic symptoms of multiple sclerosis.

Like Parkinson's, MS is one of the great neurological mysteries. The odds of a randomly selected couple like ourselves having each member contract one of these neurological conditions is minute. However, the fact that Esther's father had both spondylitis and Graves' disease, a chronic thyroid condition, and that Esther also had Graves', significantly increased the probability of her contracting multiple sclerosis. But we did not know that at the time of her diagnosis.

The only knowledge of MS that I had, other than the story of Esther's aunt, was that a friend's wife had died of it about a dozen years earlier. Now I had to learn.

Multiple sclerosis is a condition of the body's central nervous systems. It occurs when the myelin, a protective sheath around the spinal cord and the nerve fibres in the brain are eaten away, rather like an electrical wire without insulation. The nerve fibres are so densely packed that when the brain's electric current is traveling along the nerve fibres it can short out like an electrical circuit. Which parts of the body are affected depends on which circuits are compromised by the demyelination process. It is principally a young person's medical condition. Most patients develop the condition by their early twenties. Looking back, I now realize that the first signs of Esther's multiple sclerosis probably came in the early 1980s with her drooping face. There are three types of MS: Esther's is chronic progressive, which means that she does not recover from an exacerbation in a "two steps forward, one step back" fashion. The condition just steadily gets worse.

After absorbing the news of the diagnosis we realized that we had to tell Howard and Emily. We were determined not to repeat the mistake we had made after I received my diagnosis, which was to keep them in the dark. Howard was attending Lakehead University while Emily was doing her final year of high school year at the Lycée Canadienne en France. We phoned Howard and got him at his apartment. He took the news with equanimity and sympathy. With Emily it was much harder. The only number we had was the school number and she was called out of her English class—they were going over Dylan Thomas's "Do Not Go Gentle into that Good Night." Emily fought back tears as she spoke to us. We cried too. Her class turned into a support group for her that day, bonds of friendship with some have lasted to this day.

Dr. Macdonald's diagnosis was just that, a diagnosis. It didn't make Esther's condition any better or worse. But we now knew, and had to accept, that in the long run, we would have to cope with more and more difficult conditions. In the meantime, all we could do was continue living our lives as best we could.

There were practical considerations. Would Esther continue as a Trustee? She cared deeply about the issues and realized that if she resigned she would likely be replaced by someone from the socialist NDP, a possibility that she and I viewed with horror. Apart from the question of who would succeed her, there was the salary of approximately $50,000 (one third of it tax free), which was very important to our welfare, and which would end if she resigned.

In the month following the telephone diagnosis, Esther had increasing difficulty walking. She got progressively worse as Christmas approached. We were both very concerned. Parkinson's had advanced a fair bit in me, to the extent that I couldn't walk without a cane for several hours each day, and sometimes not even then. Just before Christmas, when the children would be coming home, Esther called Dr. Macdonald's office to tell him of her inability to walk. She was concerned about the children's reaction to coming home and finding that neither parent was mobile. Over the telephone, Prednisone was prescribed. It is a steroid drug which is supposed to moderate inflammation. It provided some relief, but produced internal bleeding as a side effect. Over the phone, another drug was prescribed to deal with the internal bleeding. Not for the first time, I was very concerned with the quality of medical care Esther was receiving.

In January 1993, Esther saw Dr. Trevor Gray. He had been highly recommended by the friend whose wife had died of MS in 1981. He confirmed the diagnosis, although with less enthusiasm than Dr. Macdonald had done. As Esther recovered from the attack of paraplegia, which we wanted to treat as a one-time occurrence, we both tried to imagine how she could adjust to living with MS. I felt she would have to deliberately conserve her energy and lead a quieter life. If she adopted a routine and followed it, it could make a real difference. But that was not easy to do as a school trustee.

She had taken a leave of absence from the middle of December until the end of January to get over the paraplegia and to try to get used to the idea of having MS as a life-long companion. While I tried to be supportive, my Parkinson's was progressing fairly quickly, so I wound up being resentful that I had to share the limelight of sympathy and understanding. I am ashamed now to realize that it was quite a long time, and a change in my own circumstances, before I really began caring for Esther properly. I was very good at laying down regimes for Esther to conserve herself that, I now have to acknowledge, were really designed to help her care for me.

At my next appointment with Dr. Lang, the first thing he said after hearing the news of Esther's diagnosis was a compassionate, "We have a duty to keep you mobile as long as possible." He went on to say that there were a number of options for me, including surgery.

It was a positive approach that I appreciated, but I was not emotionally ready for surgery yet. Was he out of his mind? There was no way I was going to let anyone muck around in my brain. I was beginning to think that there actually was some good stuff up there. After all, my head was a size eight and a quarter and I had always had trouble getting a hat to fit. And everyone knew of someone, or at least knew a story of someone, who had been totally screwed up by neurosurgeons.

One thing I was not being considered for was the then-current great hope for some Parkinsonians, a fetal transplant. The theory was that adrenal glands from aborted human fetuses could be placed in the brain, implanted, and that they would grow and replace the dead dopamine cells in the brain. This raised difficult moral and practical problems regarding the availability of fetuses. The spectre of "fetal harvest" has led to fascinating research on porcine fetuses, growth factors, and several other innovative approaches to what is essentially a surgical method of dopamine replacement therapy. While some progress has been made on the technology of transplantation, the fact remains that fetal transplants are significantly less successful in percentage terms than surgery involving lesions of brain tissue or brain electrical circuitry.

After Esther and I began to adjust to the news of her diagnosis, we realized that we had to face the question of how and where we should live. We had been in our house on Belsize Drive in North Toronto for sixteen years, and we liked it. Our preference was to expand it so that Esther and I and the children, who were now fully grown, could continue to live there and to renovate it so that Esther with her MS and I with my Parkinson's could more easily move around in it. The two could combine in an awesome synergy if, for example, Esther had a period when she needed assistance walking that coincided with one of the off periods for my medications; we would both be immobilized and neither able to help the other. We explained this to John Vanstone, our friend and architect. I strongly resisted the idea of "grab-rails," saying that I did not need them, but I realized that at least we had to make the house barrier free, that is, fully accessible to a disabled person, if we were to continue living there. John's first design seemed too expensive, so the summer of 1992 was spent looking at condominiums, duplexes and the resale market in houses. Those alternatives were no better, so we were back to considering a renovation.

In the previous two years, my mother had died and I had settled her estate, and my two aunts had died leaving me William Boyne's literary estate and the massive collection of prints and engravings that he had accumulated. As a result, I inherited bequests that eased our financial position, enabling us to proceed with the renovation.

Our first idea had been that the house would be extended by eight feet, which would enhance the kitchen and dining room and give more space on the second floor. We wound up gutting the whole house—the living room was the only room that wasn't structurally altered—and added approximately one thousand square feet. We extended the back of the house on the basement, first and second floors. We went far beyond just making it barrier-free. It was to be a total renovation. We had to move out of the house for ten weeks in December, January, and February while the construction was at its busiest and most frantic.

On a friend's advice we took the kitchen, main floor powder room and upstairs bathroom away from our contractor and gave the job to Chris and Gord Smith. They are artists—Gord is one of Canada's leading sculptors and Chris is involved in installation art—but they are talented artisans as well. The results were spectacular. All three rooms are barrier-free, yet you would not know it to look at them.

One thing that Esther's diagnosis had convinced us to do was to install an elevator running from the basement to the second floor, with stops at every level, including the driveway. Dr. Polak convinced us. "What would happen to your mobility if you sprained or broke an ankle? You would have a big problem. Put the elevator in."

We moved back into the house about the middle of February.

One of the first things we noticed was that one of the small drawers in Esther's dresser was missing. We then found that all of her good jewellery was missing. It was quite old and valuable, most of it handed down to us from either her family or mine. We then realized that the drawer had been stolen too—to carry the jewellery in—as had a telephone and a new fax machine not even out of its box.

The police came; then the insurance adjuster and finally the cheque, which inevitably only covered a fraction of the loss. Over the course of the next two years we discovered, indeed still are discovering, the true extent of what was stolen. We have concluded that the robbery was not a quick "grab and run"; rather it was well-organized over time. In our innocence, we trusted everyone, from family to casual workers to our contractor and his crew. We do not know to this day who was responsible for the robbery.

In retrospect, we had picked the worst imaginable time to renovate. Both Esther and I had a total lack of energy, so things were not packed away as they should have been. Fortunately, our silver was stored at a friend's house. We could not have been thinking very clearly or we would have emptied the house and put everything in storage. But we didn't.

The stress of the renovation was ongoing, for the painter and landscapers weren't gone until mid-June. It is one thing to plan a renovation; it is quite another to make it work. We set about that by scouring design magazines and hiring a young interior designer to give us ideas. I took charge of the design because Esther was so depressed and preoccupied by MS. Actually, she probably realized how much of our capital was being consumed by the renovation.

Fast on the heels of discovering the robbery, we decided to make a big change in our life. We sold our car. Earlier in 1992, I had begun to have the feeling that my driving was degenerating. Several people had told Esther, under a cloak of anonymity, that I should stop driving. I paid little heed to them, partly because I wanted to keep on driving. Only one friend, Bruce Marshall, had the courage to risk our friendship and tell me directly that I should not drive. "You are a menace on the road, Bill. For your own safety and that of others, you have got to stop driving." I was initially annoyed with him for saying that, but I slowly appreciated his directness. He was right. My decision was not even based on accidents, although there had been a few small ones. I simply decided not to drive any more because, even in my eyes, I was no longer safe on the road.

Now, for driving purposes, Esther was declared blind. She had seen her eye doctor and was stunned when he said, "Mrs. Harshaw, I must ask you to turn in your driver's licence." While Esther had not been driving for some time, the shock of having her licence actually taken away was immense.

We had to learn to live with and, as best we could, enjoy the consequences of our limitations. Shannon Graham and Dianne Vanstone, the wives of my friends Tony, and John started taking me shopping—to the St. Lawrence Market, the Price Club, Loblaws, and so on. It was fun and I remarked at Esther's 1993 birthday party that I saw more of their wives than they did!

Learning to accept the help of friends was one of the lessons we had to learn. Learning not to depend on that help and not to take it for granted was another. I came to realize that I was using my friends as my personal support group. I hadn't gone to them and asked, "will you help me cope with Parkinson's by being my support group?" They just offered of their own accord: Stephen Booth, Ian Hamilton, Howard Shill, Tony Graham, and a number of others. What I did not think about at that time was that there are many Parkinsonians who do not have a supportive family or group of friends.

During the most intense period of the renovation, from November through February, we had moved out of the house and into the Royal York Hotel. It might seem a lavish alternative but in fact it was practical—the hotel offered us an attractive rate, and we needed the services it could provide. My Parkinson's had been progressing rapidly, with violently contrasting moments of akinesia and dyskinesia depending on whether my meds were on or off. Esther's MS had led to an attack of paraplegia. At Christmas, Howie and Emily, back from their schools, stayed at the hotel as well and saw us at our worst. A cousin of Esther's, Nell West, also stayed with us over Christmas.

One evening, when neither Esther nor I could walk very well, we were on our way to dinner in the hotel dining room. Our movement was slow and hesitating. We must have looked like old people in young bodies. Esther could be pulled forward; sometimes when I couldn't walk forward I could walk backwards. I put my arms around Esther, and said in my best Yul Brynner voice, "Shall we dance?" And dance we did, in a fashion, to the imaginary orchestra playing the Rogers and Hammerstein tune from The King and I until we arrived at our table to the bemused looks of patrons and restaurant staff. Much to my surprise and embarrassment, they applauded us, not because we looked like Fred Astaire and Ginger Rogers, but because we got there on our own.

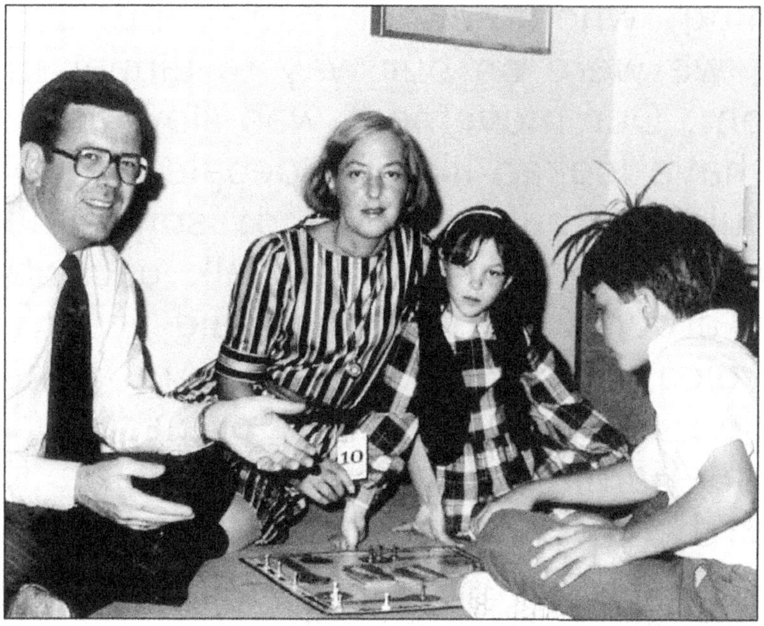

The Harshaws—Me, Esther, Emily, and Howie—in 1981, before Parkinson's.

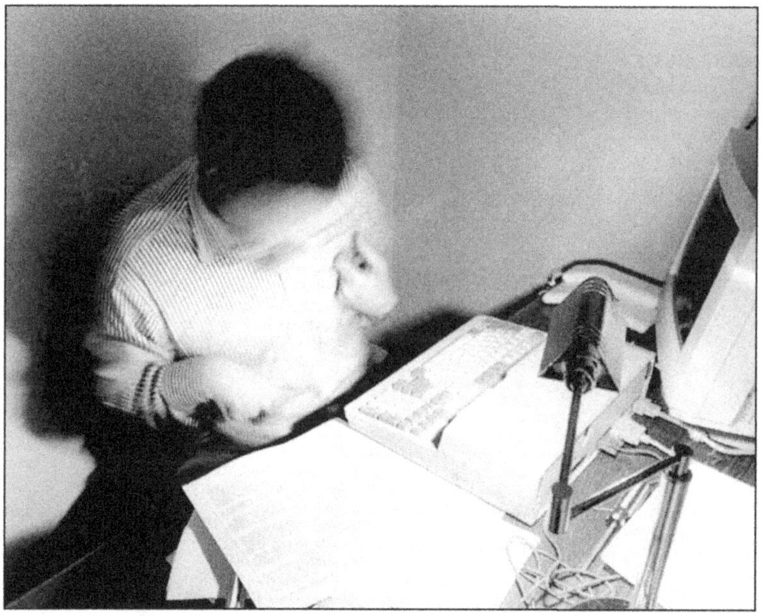

When my dyskinesias (a side effect of medication) were at their worst, just before my first operation in 1993.

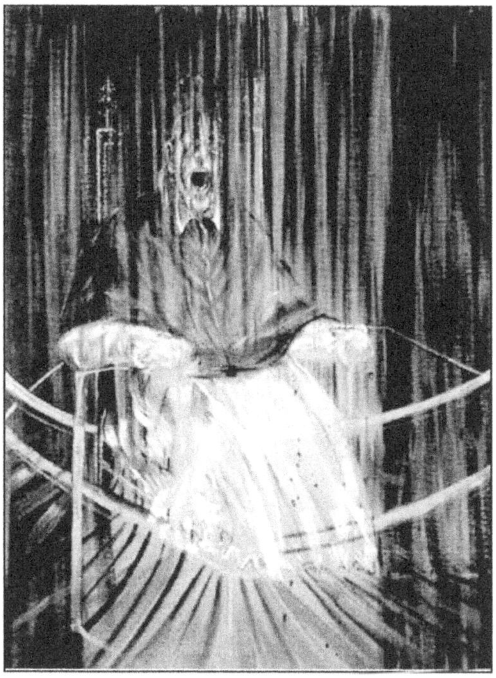

Before my first operation in 1993, when my condition was at its worst, I felt the agony portrayed in Francis Bacon's Study after Velásquez's Portrait of Pope Innocent X, the supreme modern representation of anguish and powerlessness

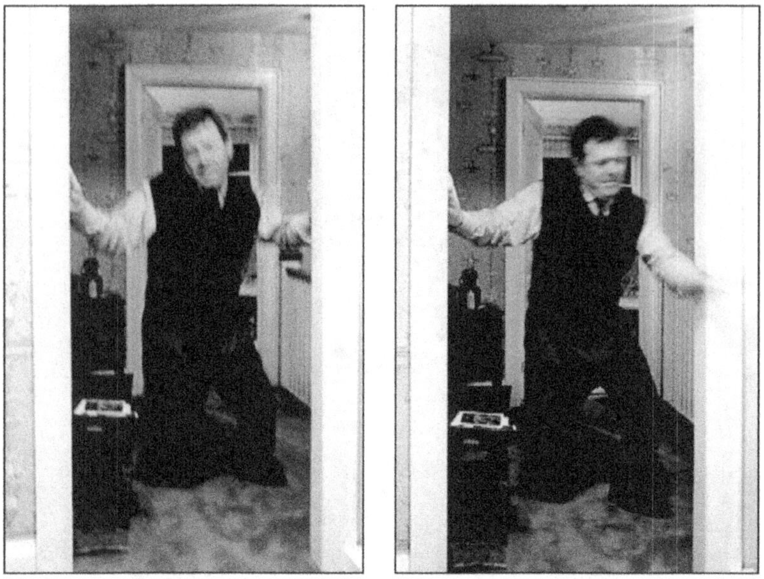

When my medications were "off," moving from one room to another required a major effort.

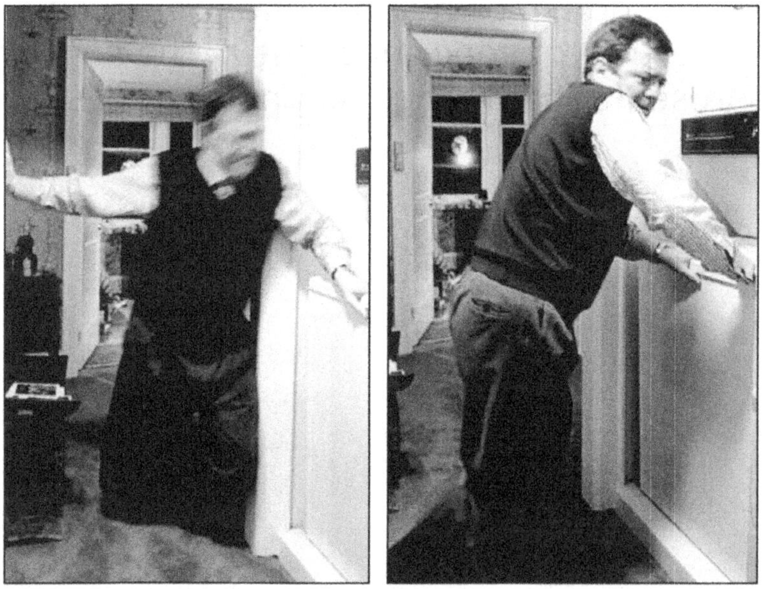

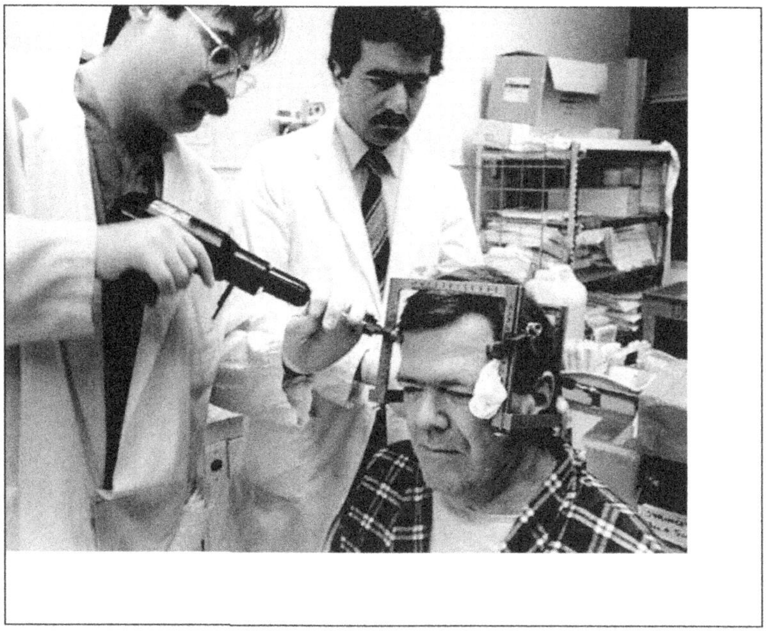

A combination of high tech and home toolbox: securing the stereotactic frame with a Black and Decker™ cordless drill. The driller is Dr. Michael Munz, a Neurosurgical Fellow; observing is a visiting doctor from Turkey.

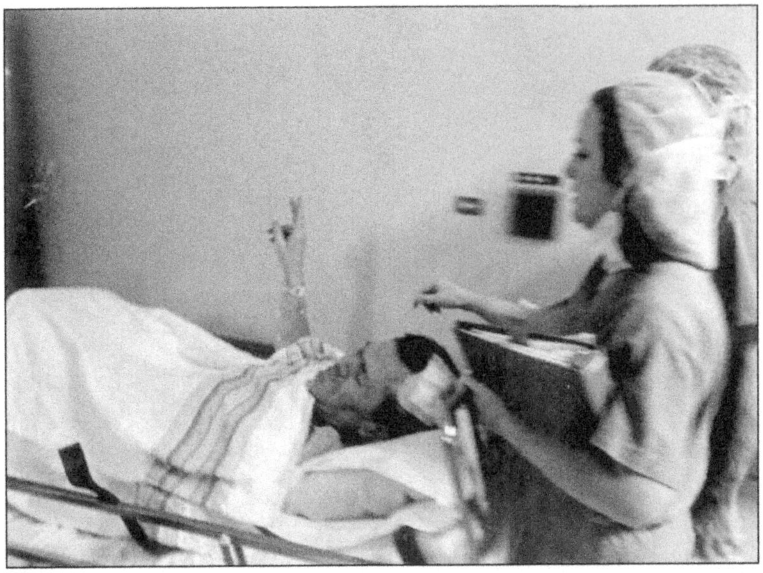

Just after the second operation, on the way to the Recovery Room. Right hand raised in a "V" for victory over Parkinson's disease.

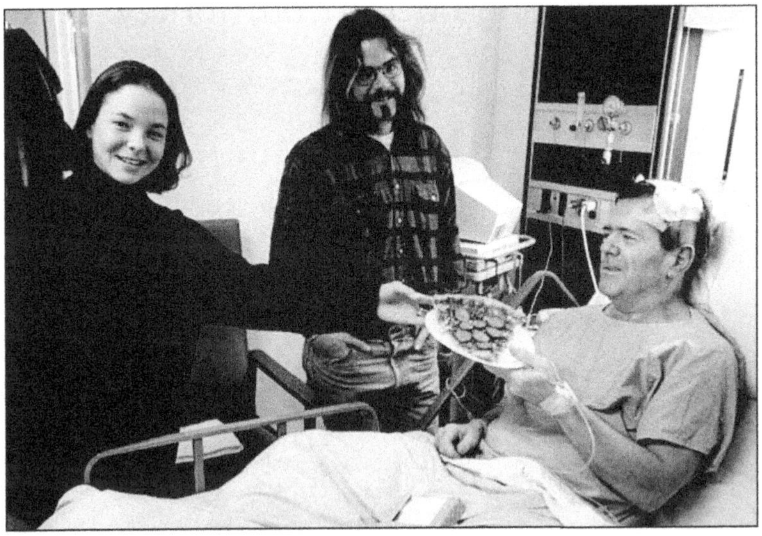

Eating a pizza after the second operation with Emily and Howie.

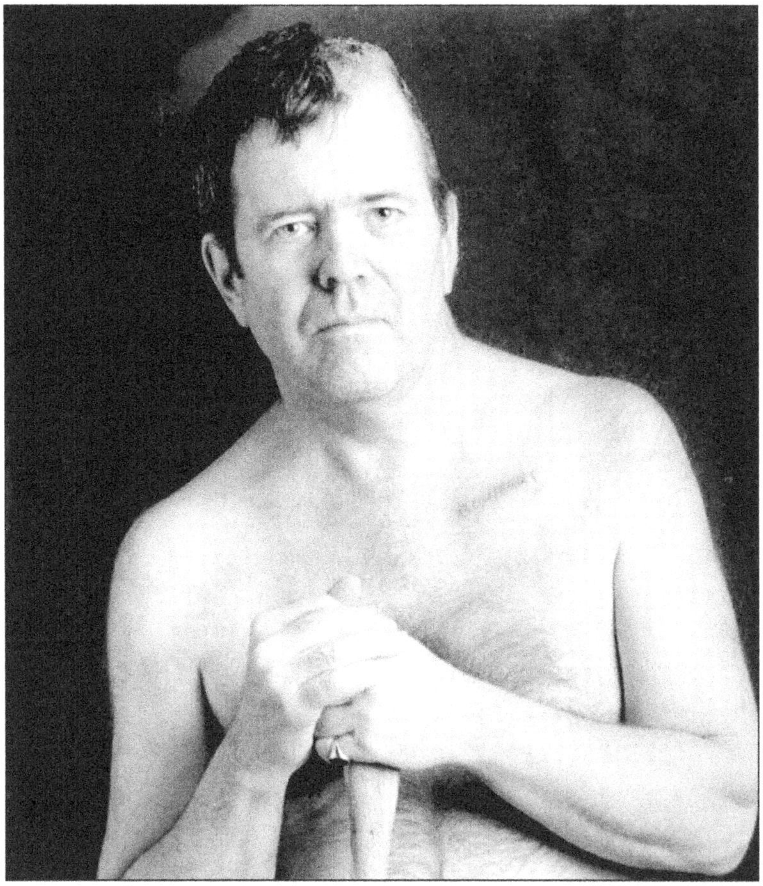

The bare me after the second operation. Note the stapled incision on my left collarbone where my neurostimulator is implanted. The bald spot is where the electrodes enter my brain.

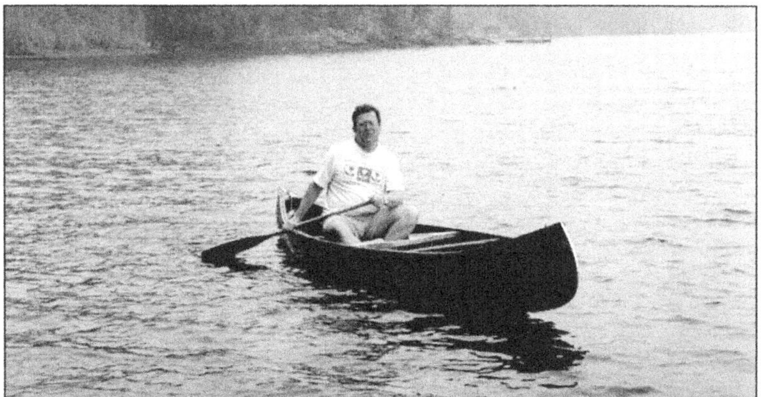

Enjoying a solitary paddle in my canoe at Blue Sea Lake.

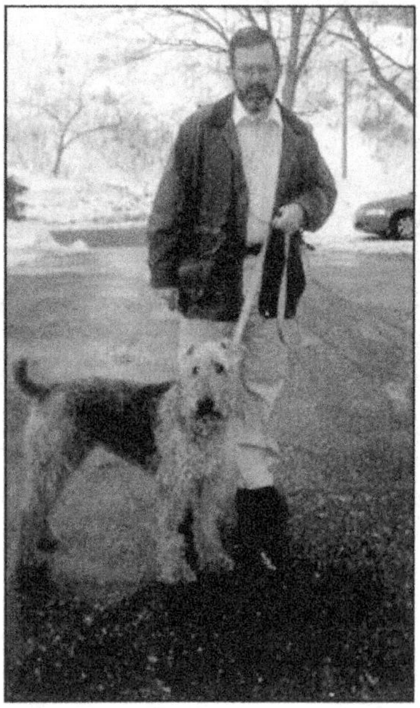

With Madam in January 2001.

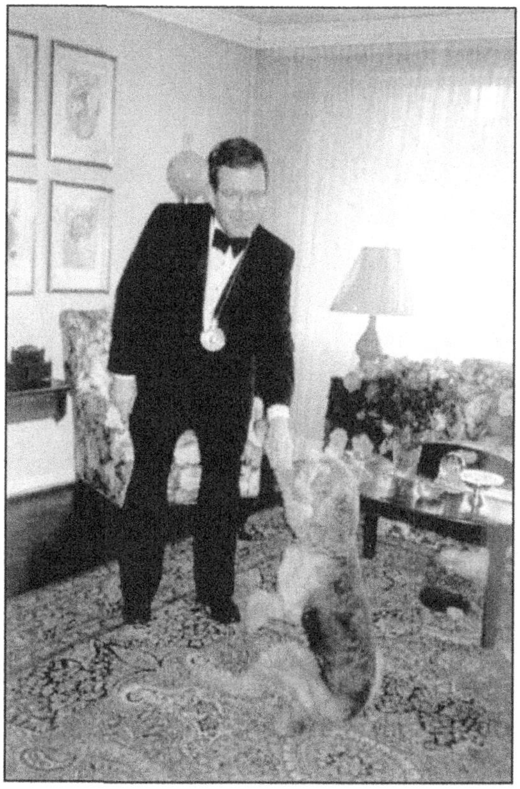

Madam and me, formal.

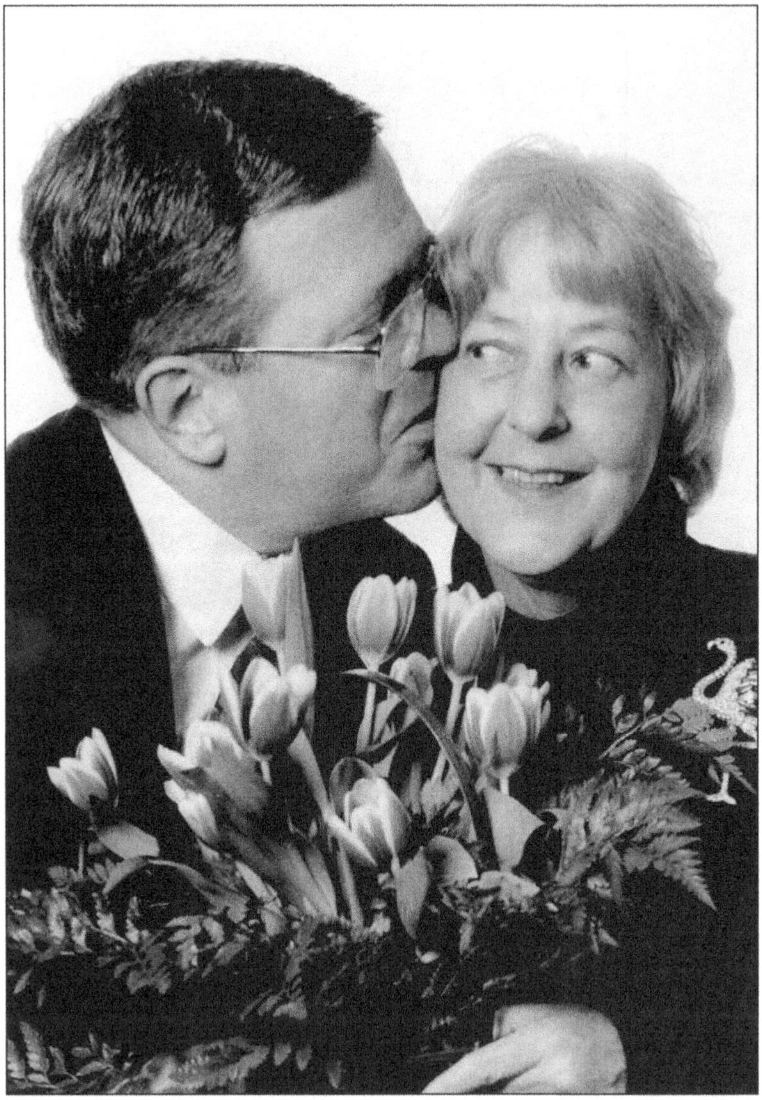

Esther and me in March, 1996

CHAPTER SEVEN

Advent

Mornings were a dull routine.
Immobile.
Many hours would pass until my brain's command
My anxious limbs its tortured message reached.
And permitted steps, first halting
Like a child would take.
Then runstumble.
Strangers asked:
"What troubles him?
His legs like branches on a misshaped tree
Do move in deformed harmony

*****

I was walking along Yonge Street in Toronto one day in the summer of 1993. Some passers-by would give me an unusual look, some a frightened, uncertain stare; a few even crossed over to the other side of the street. They felt threatened by the contortions of my upper body. I was writhing uncontrollably, like some sort of primitive reptile and my face was distorted, mask-like. My walking was distinctly irregular, with both legs limping and dragging and I seemed almost incapacitated. I looked like an escapee from Wanless's freak show, which Robertson Davies so effectively described in his novel, World of Wonders. My speech was slurred and rushed as if I was drunk. To people who encountered me I seemed to be incomprehensible, probably a lunatic, possibly dangerous.

I didn't fully realize that this was how most people saw me until a dinner party we had with the Van Straubenzees and the Grahams in December. I gave a dramatic reading of one of the short stories I had been writing over the past few years, and Tony Graham videotaped my performance on our camcorder. I was shocked at the result.

For the first time I realized how grotesque and freak-like I was in appearance. Parkinson's had really disfigured me. I was abnormal. The contortions of my face and body were more like a person with cerebral palsy, but without the internal harmony and rhythm that characterizes that neurological affliction. My face had become an immobile reptilian mask. It was devastating to me. The tormented apocalyptic visions that William Blake and John Martin had portrayed in their nineteenth century engravings did not come close to the way I saw myself. What I felt was more akin to the agony portrayed in Francis Bacon's Study after Velásquez's Portrait of Pope Innocent X, the supreme modern representation of anguish and powerlessness. And the irony of Parkinson's, for me at least, is that the anguish is emotional—I have never endured significant physical pain.

Did I rage against God? Not exactly, although I asked why both Esther and I were afflicted with incurable neurological diseases. I raged against Man. Who, specifically, did I rage against? The editors at ABC for lack of editorial direction, the duplicity of my independent editorial readers, and the thieves who robbed our house while the renovation was going on, to name just three that come immediately to mind. I raged against anyone and anything that seemed to be against me, who treated me condescendingly. I raged and railed against them as examples of the bad things in God's creation. Pretty immature and trivial compared to some of the world's great human tragedies. As humanity is made in the imagination of God, I got angry at God's limited imagination.

Here is a poem I wrote during these months that conveyed something of what I was feeling.

LAZARUS

I

The day began normally for me
Up at five. Run.
At seven leave.
Drive there on the 401.
Arrive shaking from the tension
of driving. Or so I thought.
Until the doctor said:
"Parkinson's." Esther cried.

The doctor said:
"You will be able to tie flies again."
The fool had no sense of what's important

Nor had I.
I tried to hide the shaking hand,
the dragging foot.
To no avail. One day I said:
"No, not hangover. Parkinson's."

No pain
No movement
No work.
Pension at forty five.

A baker's dozen years now
I raged like Sampson.
I did not curse God
I tried to understand
Why me?
There is no reason.
There never is.
So, why not me?

It is perverse.
Some days I move at will
Others cannot despite my will.

It moves in leaps as if to curb
My pleasure.
I am trapped inside my body

But not in prison.
For I have much to do before I go;
I must complete the task
Fulfil the vision

II

There are others who do not know
Why they are different,
Or what makes them so.
They live in squalor and
Fear
Of what they do not know.

Because we are indifferent
Because we care more for the far away
Than the near
Bosnia, not Regent's Park
New neighbourhoods to us
Xenophobia is powerful
We are afraid of what we do not know.

The Good Samaritan shared not our cares
He helped without reward.
We have neither
Soul nor imagination.
We care what others think
Emotion does not show.
It is unmanly
To stop before satiety
Or so we think.

He said: "The poor are always with us.
"Do not make Him a liar,
For He is Perfect
And cannot lie.

We are our brother's keeper.
Providence keeps us.
We defy it hedonically
Always testing limits
We are the hollow men
and do not know it.
We whimper at affronts to comfort
And repeat old words
That cleanse guilt
Like silver polish
No effort.

III

We go about from day to day
Seeing nothing but footsteps,
Smelling only the ordinary and execrable
Feeling nothing but kitchen textures and
Bedroom emotions.
What closes our eyes to wonder/
Our touch to the exquisite?
The mind to the unknown?

Why are we afraid to explore the beyond?
Examine the rose without thought of time
Or consequence

Shut off all around.
Let concentration become meditation
Surrounded by what was always there
Now understood.

Creation transforms us
I we let it, into
New people freed of the opaquing caul
that clouds the senses
numbs the mind

IV

We do not think
of disability
When we are young.
We will be forever young.
Perfection
we look for and find not

Now half the time
I cannot walk
Cannot write
Speech is slurred.
I can see and
Hear
And touch.

Pain is transient.
It is easy to sit and
Not initiate ... anything.

People understand that it is hard.
The anguish of a song unsung,
A book unwritten is as impotence
To creation. We are free to choose.

We become the passive people
Beneficiaries of goodwill expressed
Without asking us
What, when, where...
We would like...
No matter ... they know best
We only have PD,
The object of their charity

I am Lazarus
There are gradations of Hell
I know them all.
I am not a survivor
I am the strongest and best.
I must be
To endure Hell.
I am Lazarus
I am not chosen
I have made the choice
to be free.

Parkinson's had progressed in me in the past year to the stage where I was now immobile, trapped, for half the waking day. During the other half, I needed help walking, usually using two sticks. There were short periods when I could walk unaided, but these were unreliable. Without medication I could not move at all and had to be in a wheelchair. Dyskinesia, a side effect of L-dopa medications, had become a real problem. The radius of my upper body movement was two and a half feet (80 centimetres for metric types). If I were in a China shop, I would be a bull.

My appearance and slurred speech, which did not reflect anything I felt physically or emotionally, were extremely off-putting to others, particularly people who did not know me, and alienating for me. The neurologist and writer, Oliver Sacks, gives a vivid description of one of his patients that applied well to me.

> ...he would sometimes speak of his body as a prison, with windows but no doors. He also saw himself as being exiled from proper life and from other people...[5]

The principal anti-Parkinsonian medications—Sinemet CR and Prolopa effectively moderate Parkinsonian symptoms of immobility but they also cause dyskinesia as a side effect. As dosage rises and the length of time the patient uses the medication increases, the side effects become worse. The physician, working with the patient, looks for an acceptable compromise.

By this time, I was taking fourteen Sinemet CR tablets daily, well over the usual maximum recommended dosage. But I was faced with a Hobson's choice: to increase the dosage to the extent necessary to make me fully mobile, in which case the accompanying dyskinesia would be incapacitating; or to reduce the dosage to the extent required to eliminate dyskinesia in which case I would be immobilized.

Despite the horror I felt at the video film of my reading at our dinner party, I actually had a reason to hope that my condition might be improved. Earlier that year, in April, Dr. Lang had suggested that I consider experimental neurosurgery as a partial alternative to drug therapy. He recognized that mobility was a real priority for me because of the implications of Esther's condition. He explained that the surgery was not a cure for Parkinson's, but would be an interim solution to my declining drug response rate. The medications were simply becoming less effective, increasingly going off at random during the day for periods of time varying from half an hour to three or four hours, leaving me immobilized.

The proposed operation, a pallidotomy, involves making a lesion, or scar tissue, on the globus pallidus, the part of the brain that regulates movement. To make the lesions, the surgeon would have to make precise, minute probes through my skull into the brain. The probe would then be heated and burn a tiny part of the brain tissue that was producing the difficulties in movement in my body. This surgery, if successful, could ease the symptoms, meaning a lower dosage of the drugs could provide me with the same or better relief. I had resisted the idea at first, but as the summer wore on I became increasingly attracted to it.

The Toronto Western Hospital has one of, if not the, largest and best assembly of neuroscience professionals in North America, ranging from nurse practitioners and general neurologists to sub-specialist neurologists and neurosurgeons who are world leaders in their field of specialization. It doesn't stop there. Support specialists, such as neuro-pathologists, neuro-radiologists, and sub-sub-specialists—neuro-gastroenterologists, for example—round out this galaxy of stars that make the Western the premier neuroscience site in Canada

Even our idyllic holiday at Blue Sea Lake had its frustrations. We have been staying with Nell West since Esther's sister Mary and her husband Tony bought the big cottage on the hill. Nell is Esther's cousin and has been to me like the sister I never had. She has been totally and unreservedly accepting of me as Parkinson's steadily progresses through my body. She is a V.O.N. nurse and is very familiar with Parkinson's—probably more than she would like to be—and with multiple sclerosis. It was her mother, Esther West, the twin sister of my Esther's mother, who had had MS. Nell's laid-back manner is very deceptive: it conceals a love of fun and parties as well as detailed knowledge of what is and is not important in the scheme of things. These were qualities that Esther and I came to appreciate more and more as our conditions developed.

Nell's cottage had an inadequate septic field that couldn't absorb a full summer's use. Consequently we used the outhouse as much as possible. I was determined to co-operate and used it all the time, even when it made no sense to do so. When it was pouring rain for instance. One night I woke up at about 3a.m. and tried to make it to the outhouse, even though my meds were off and I could hardly move. It was a combination of bullheadedness and sheer stupidity. I stumbled and fell; no damage was done, except to my pride. After all, if you cannot go to the bathroom on your own, you're in pretty rough shape. Anger and frustration welled up in me. I was at the end of my tether.

When I got back in the cottage, I stumbled to my bedroom, got a cheque, made it out to Nell, and signed it, leaving the amount blank. I had made quite a commotion, so Esther and Nell were awake and were worried about me, wondering if I had hurt myself. I brushed aside their questions and shouted: "Take this cheque and fix the bloody septic field so it can be used all summer long. I damn near killed myself out there."

They both started crying. "Bill", said Nell, "we were worried about you; you could have hurt yourself badly."

It was an emotional scene. I realized slowly how stupid I had been, taking such a high risk to satisfy my stubborn pride. I had to face the fact that I was disabled, nearly crippled.

During the summer my condition continued to deteriorate and I was being tried on liquid Sinemet, in the form of a cocktail comprising Tang, ascorbic acid, and Sinemet 100/10 and water. This was supposed to be absorbed into the system more quickly by taking pills, and therefore to cross the blood/brain barrier more quickly. Only it didn't in my case.

In late August I described my condition in a letter to Dr. Lang.

> During the course of the last month, both walking and dyskinesia have deteriorated to the extent that my waking hours are, on an average day, more off than on, notwithstanding attempts to regulate walking with regular Sinemet. I suspect its use makes dyskinesia worse.
>
> Two weeks ago, Jan phoned to ask if I would be interested in an experimental neurosurgery procedure which could have the effect of improving walking and permit a reduction in drug dosages. My answer then was "yes". Now, with the experience of the last couple of weeks, my "yes" is even stronger. Esther and I have discussed it as far as we can without my having discussed the procedure and the probabilities with the surgeon. I look forward to his call.

In August, Jan Duff, Dr. Lang's clinical trials co-ordinator, gave me a date for surgery, October 27, and said that I would have to come to the hospital for baseline testing about two weeks before. The idea behind the tests was to have a benchmark against which the doctors could measure my post-surgical performance. One aspect made me very apprehensive: I would have to go off my medications for about twelve hours. I would probably be completely incapacitated and would see more fully than I could bear how far Parkinson's disease had progressed in me, and how utterly dependent I was on drug therapy. I should not have worried about that. For a period of time in early October there was doubt about my making it to the starting gate, to say nothing of winning the race.

At about this time, the subject of assisted suicide was very much in the public eye. It was an approach to which I strongly objected. A British Columbia woman with terminal multiple sclerosis who wished to end her own life had carried on a campaign with dignity. At about the same time, Erwhin Krickhaln, a patient with a chronic and terminal neurological condition (and who was a pathetic individual to boot) carried on his campaign with all the hype and dignity of a circus freak-show and received a lot of publicity. He proposed selling his story and admitting certain member of the press to witness his assisted suicide. A article sympathetic to Krickhaln and the subject of assisted suicide appeared in The Globe and Mail. A letter of reply I wrote to the editor was subsequently published.

> A private act has been turned into a public spectacle ... Death is the last act of our temporal lives. With the abolition of public executions in the nineteenth century, even criminals were allowed to die in privacy. What right does Mr. Krickhaln have to impose the act of his death on the public?
>
> At this point may I say that I have some knowledge of the manner in which neuro-degenerative diseases affect those that have them. I am 50 and have had Parkinson's disease for 13 years. My mobility becomes more constrained with each passing day. For about half my waking hours I cannot walk unassisted if at all, and my situation is not unique. I do not despair. I have never contemplated killing myself. Nor do most men and women with complex neurological diseases.
>
> Articles like this one do a grave disservice to the thousands of men and women who do not let their diseases defeat them; who with little more than their own initiative to guide them surmount the obstacles their diseases place in front of them. Indeed, articles such as Sean Fine's could give newly diagnosed patients the impression that suicide is the preferred course of action in the

> long term. Nothing could be farther from the truth. Courage and determination have not been tried and found wanting. They have been found difficult and left untried.

My views on assisted suicide haven't really altered in the years since the article and my letter were written. I still feel it is giving up on life at a time when the prospects seem utterly bleak. I am an optimist. The American surgeon Sherwin B. Nuland, in his wonderful book, How We Live, expresses the point very well:

> A disease presents itself in a unique form in each person it attacks, and it pursues a unique course. Every good or bad prognosis is a statement of probability, not of fact.... Whether the number appear favourable or foul, the outcome of your or my sickness is ultimately decided by unknown factors within us. They will probably remain unknowable for decades or even centuries to come, if not forever.

In our society, the emerging consensus is increasingly in favour of permitting assisted suicide for patients in narrowly defined terminal situations. But I think the opposing views should continue to be heard.

My letter to The Globe and Mail shows, as clearly as anything can, the extent to which I had turned the tables on Parkinson's. It no longer ran my life. In fact, despite the many frustrations, I was becoming almost manic in my approach to life, feeling there was so much I wanted to do—no, felt I must do.

My biography of Archbishop Clark was close to completion. Ted Scott had discussed the final draft with a quartet of editorial readers: Stephen Booth, Eugene Fairweather, Michael Hicks, and Barry Valentine. Editorial changes were made and the final draft was sent to the Anglican Book Centre. Its response was delivered to me second-hand from Bishop Jack Bothwell, who was readying a book of his own for publication by the ABC: "Tell Harshaw that he might want to leave a copy of his manuscript with General Synod Archives."

On the delivery of that insult, I determined to publish the book myself. As I quickly learned, there is more to publishing a book than just paying the printer's bill. There is typesetting, design, distribution to be arranged, publicity, International Standard Book Numbers ... the list seemed endless. All these things had to be done in October and November if I wanted the book out in December. Friends pitched in. Julian Porter helped with choosing the printer, my account manager at Scotiabank played a key role in negotiating the contract with the printer, Pete Paterson organized the photographs and the layout and Joyce Hamilton designed the book and the cover.

That summer, 1993, I found myself again reminded of how ineffectual Parkinson's was rendering me. I had been a member of Synod, the governing body of the Anglican Diocese of Toronto, for over twenty years. The 1993 session was controversial, in part due to me. I wanted to raise a constitutional issue: on a vote would "refused ballots" be counted as cast ballots or spoiled ballots? A refused ballot is one taken by an voter, and immediately turned back to the scrutineer unmarked. Traditionally, in Anglican Church procedure, refused ballots were treated as spoiled ballots and not counted. In civil politics, at all three levels of government, they are treated as cast ballots and are counted. I believed this principle should apply to votes at Synod. As I am a Bishop's appointee to Synod, I informed him and the Chancellor, the chief legal officer, of my intention to ask that refused ballots be counted as cast ballots. I did not want to blindside either one of them.

Rising (that's an ironic turn of phrase—"Slowly and haltingly got up" would be better) on a point of privilege, I gave my speech in an almost inaudible voice, rushing my words together. I felt embarrassed. My point would be lost. and what was more important to me, the world, or at least the members of Synod, could see how incapacitated I had become. The Bishop came to my rescue, asking the Chancellor to read my remarks, which I had typed out. He read my statement perfunctorily and then dismissed my request as inappropriate.

Stephen Booth asked, "Is that a ruling?"

The Bishop nodded to the Chancellor. The Chancellor replied, "Yes, My Lord."

A second priest asked: "Is the ruling subject to appeal?"

The Bishop nodded again.

"No!" said the Chancellor.

At a break in the session, friends congratulated me in taking what was bound to be an unpopular stand against the Bishop. Nonetheless, I was still humiliated; I felt I had been patronized by the Bishop and Chancellor because of my Parkinsonian disability.

During this summer and autumn, Esther was in comparatively good shape. The serious MS attack she had the previous December had abated and she was now back to being a school trustee, albeit at a slower pace than before. She told her colleagues and others that she was "temporarily otherly-abled."

On the last Sunday in September, just a month before my scheduled operation, I staged a lunch for my dining club, the Alderbrandin de Sienne Society. Esther had an appointment the next day with an MS specialist in Buffalo, so she wasn't there—Gillian Booth acted as hostess. Eighteen for lunch—I would be testing myself even if I did not have Parkinson's. The menu was melon soup, leg of lamb, and a cold Grand Marnier soufflé and the wines were an '89 Ockfener Bechstein Auslese, '80 Romanée Saint Vivant, and '76 Reisling Beerenauslese. I did all the cooking, but hired two maids to help serve. The eighteen of us sat at the dining room table and at two bridge tables. The lunch went well—indeed, all went well. There were leftovers of everything and I took them over to John and Dianne Vanstone's for dinner. It was a perfect day. I had pulled off the lunch party!

I woke up at 2:00a.m. the next morning with no strength in my left side at all. "Shit!... have I had a stroke?" was my first thought. I made it to the bathroom, which was why I had wakened, and back to bed with great difficulty. I can't have taken the idea of a stroke very seriously because I got back to sleep in no time. When I woke up in the morning, about a third of my strength had returned. I fussed and fumed all morning trying to decide whether or not to tell the doctors. I was afraid the incident would lead to postponing or canceling the operation. I finally did the responsible thing and called Dr. Polak at noon; about half my strength had returned. He saw me at 3p.m. by which time about 75 percent of my normal strength had returned to my left side.

Dr. Polak examined me thoroughly but could find no explanation for what had happened. He then diagnosed it as transitory selective muscle weakness (I later learned that is what they call something when they don't know what causes it), and assured me that there were no implications for my pending operation. "But, I'll phone Tony Lang and let him know." That was on Monday. Lang saw me on Thursday at noon; usually it takes three months to get an appointment with him.

When he asked me to get on the examining table, I leapt up, doing a half turn in mid-air, like Baryshnikov (at least I thought I looked like him).

"Show-off" said Dr. Lang, coolly. His examination of me was comprehensive and led to one conclusion. "There's probably nothing wrong with you, but I wouldn't want you to have a stroke on the operating table. I'm putting the operation on hold pending the results of some tests you're going to have."

My fears of having my operation deferred were realized. Because of the logjam caused by the provincial government's cost-cutting "Social Contract," the tests could not be done for two weeks, and the results would not be to hand until the end of the month. And I hadn't even had my baseline tests that were to precede the operation.

Despite the delay, Providence was on my side. The tests showed there was nothing to prevent me from having the operation. The problem now lay with operating room time. The Social Contract again. This was elective surgery, i.e. it was not required to save my life. The hospital had to put elective surgery on hold. It looked like I was going to be put off until the New Year.

I did not take this lying down. On October 21, I wrote to Dr. Lang.

> I was taken aback yesterday when Jan Duff told me that I would not likely have surgery until

> January next year, a delay of at least two months; the delay being due to the Social Contract causing the hospital to close the surgeon's operating theatre for December and half of November.
>
> I am shocked and not a little depressed that, after the matter leaves your hands and enters the bureaucracy, it will take four weeks to order and get back test results, when surgery time had been booked for October 29.
>
> As well, the effect of the Social Contract on health care is a random shock that you could not have factored into your plans; I was naive enough to think "it will not effect me." I do not envy you and your colleagues as you are forced to practice triage that has a political imperative rather than a battlefield cause. Perhaps it is a different battlefield, one few of us are equipped effectively to deal with.
>
> Of course, I will manage until surgery can be scheduled. My mobility is increasingly constrained. As I write—it is now 11:15a.m.—I have been up for seven hours and will not likely be "on" until early afternoon, and then there is no guarantee how long I will be "on."

A few days later, in a moment of intense frustration, I said to Dr. Lang and Jan Duff: "If you're in line to see a movie and you leave to take a leak, when you return, you resume your place in line; you don't go to the end." My remark seemed to have the desired effect. I was booked for testing on November 8 and 9, with the operation scheduled for December 8.

On October 31, I turned 50. To celebrate, Esther had a lunch party for me on November 7. There were sixty guests. It began at 1 and ended about 5. The day gave me a real lift. The big surprise came when I was presented with a Certificate of Merit by Bishop Finlay for my service to the Church in the Diocese of Toronto.

The next day I set off to the hospital for the pre-operative testing. The procedure was exhausting but fun. Most of the time the first day was taken up with neuropsychological testing—things like word association, short-term memory, relationships between shapes, abstract thinking, and numerous other tests to establish a cognitive baseline of data against which my post-operative neuro-psych tests would be measured. A few of the answers were "non-standard," that is, they did not conform to standard responses. For instance, in a verbal association test when the word "fabric" was given, I responded "church," because it is the traditional term referring to the construction and maintenance of church buildings. The neuropsychologist who was administering this battery of tests did not know what to make of me. When the testing was completed, he consulted Dr. Jean St. Cyr, the chief of the service. St. Cyr's assessment: "Mr.

Harshaw, you are very bright, if not brilliant. You are also a bit of a smart ass." I did not demur.

I stayed overnight in hospital. The next day I was to do the neurological tests, which were what I had been most apprehensive about. They involved being off medications, so my meds were withheld from 10p.m. the evening before until Jan Duff had done the off tests on the following morning. That meant no Sinemet or Pergolide at midnight, 2:30a.m., 5a.m., and 7:30a.m., my normal nightly regimen. "Off meds": the phrase was enough to strike terror into my heart. I didn't know what it would be like but I imagined that I couldn't do anything by myself, not even pee, or brush my teeth. And it would show me how completely dependent I was on medication for what little mobility I did have.

All this was true, although the anticipation was much worse than the event. I was still terrified. As I could not move, I had to be bathed by an orderly, and eating breakfast was difficult. Jan came to get me at 8a.m. with a wheelchair. I certainly wasn't going anywhere on my own! We got up to the movement disorders clinic and the tests began. The tests, which were videotaped, included walking, standing up without assistance, balance, various tests of muscular rigidity, and a speech test. After those tests, I was scored between the eightieth and eighty-fifth percentiles. That meant only fifteen to 20 percent of Parkinsonians had worse symptoms than me. No more slow marches; Parkinson's was going through me at double time.

I was frightened by those results. If the operation wasn't successful I realized there was the likelihood that I would sooner rather than later be incarcerated in a chronic care institution, not being able to see or write, with my speech being impaired. I would be cut off from the world and the world would be cut off from me.

Esther says that I have never complained about Parkinson's. But I did my best to hide my anxiety. If I accuse Esther of being a good actress, I am guilty of the having the same skill. During the previous couple of months I had been so busy with getting my book published, and taking on new responsibilities with the Toronto Chapter of the Parkinson's Foundation that I ignored my disabilities. How long could I expect to do this?

In fact, I was so concerned with the book that Pete Paterson and I met at lunchtime on the day I was having the neuropsychological tests and he brought the layouts for the photographs over to the hospital that evening.

Later that same evening, Dr. Ronald Tasker came to see me. He was the senior functional neurosurgeon at the Western. Neurosurgeons are considered to be prima donnas in a profession where arrogance is assumed to be a sine qua non. As a group, they are probably brightest of the best, simply because the brain is the most complex organ in the human body and it is the last great frontier of medical science. I have now gotten to know three of them. Rather than arrogant, I have found them single-minded in their pursuit of understanding the brain, and singularly compassionate in their dealings with patients.

Dr. Tasker, the doyen of the very small and exclusive fraternity of functional neurosurgeons around the world, was a balding, slightly portly man wearing one of the turtleneck sweaters that were his trademark. I learned that he was a keen ornithologist.

That evening, in what I thought was a desultory sort of way, Dr. Tasker and I chatted about my upcoming pallidotomy. I later realized that his laid-back style was calculated to relax me and give him the opportunity of assessing for himself whether or not I would be a suitable candidate for the operation. Like many surgeons, Tasker felt his own judgement was a key factor. Indeed, he would book patients referred from outside the Western without the pre-op work-ups. It was not arrogance; rather it was confidence in his ability as one of the most innovative functional neurosurgeons of his generation.

My surgery date, less than a month away, was confirmed.

CHAPTER EIGHT

Neurosurgery

> ...the brain is the most interesting, complex and wonderful thing in the universe ... and it's a wonderfully exciting thing to study and be in contact with.... The brain is you, it's not just biologically or genetically, it has all your experience, it's you.
>
> -Oliver Sacks[6]

When I returned to the hospital on Tuesday, December 7, 1993, I was ready for surgery, eagerly looking forward to the operation even though I was apprehensive. Other than my overnight doing the pre-op testing I hadn't stayed in a hospital since I was twelve years old having my tonsils out, and I enjoyed the novelty. I brought a good supply of books and music tapes. Because the operation was unusual, everyone seemed to want to know about me and I was being paid a lot of attention. I felt quite important.

I was sharing a room with a man from Huntsville who had an inoperable brain tumour. His wife was with him constantly, and I sensed, from overhearing the doctors and nurses, that he did not have long to live.

Even so, there was a sense of calm surrounding the couple as they prepared for his inevitable death.

The first few hours after I was admitted were spent having my medical history taken and being visited by Jan Duff, Dr. Lang, and Esther and Howard, and so I was too busy to take in the reality of what was going on beside me. I dimly recognized that this couple was preparing for the husband's death, but there was no weeping and gnashing of teeth; rather, there was hope. As the wife left that Tuesday evening, she turned to me and said, "You will be in my prayers tonight. God bless you."

She had enough room in her heart for me, when I would have thought her whole being would be focused on her husband, on her family. I was touched and inspired by her generosity of spirit.

Later in the evening, Dr. Lozano and Dr. Tasker, the neurosurgeons, came to see me and discuss the operation. Dr. Andres Lozano is tall, with close-cropped black hair and wears plain wire-rimmed glasses. If anything, they made him look younger than his thirty-six years. He had the aura of an ascetic about him. He was the expert in pallidotomies, having done thirteen previous ones at the hospital. Dr. Tasker, with a reputation for iconoclastic brilliance, was Lozano's mentor. Tasker pioneered the thalamotomy, where lesions are made in the thalmus to relieve Parkinson's tremors. In my operation Dr. Tasker, although the senior, would be the number two surgeon, learning the pallidotomy procedure from Dr. Lozano. With me they were a "good guy, bad guy" team as they discussed the risks and potential benefits of the operation. Tasker spelled out the negatives, while Lozano emphasized the potential benefits.

The operation I would be having was a stereotaxic pallidotomy. Stereotaxic refers to the finely calibrated metal frame that would be fixed to my skull for the operation. It fulfills two functions: it provides precise three dimensional co-ordinates for the positioning of surgical instruments within the brain; and it is bolted to the operating table, immobilizing the frame, and therefore the head. The term "pallidotomy" refers to the globus pallidus, literally "pale globe," a part of the basal ganglia that is the deepest in the skull. The pallidus regulates the braking action of the brain; in Parkinson's patients the brakes are being applied too heavily, causing poverty of movement and clumsiness. (Parkinson himself had noted that sometimes, if patients of "his" disease had a stroke, the characteristic Parkinsonian tremor was less evident, although muscle weakness more than made up for the eased tremor.) In the pallidotomy, the neurosurgeons make some lesions on the pallidus that would result in scarring. When properly placed, the scars relieve the patient's symptoms.

Stereotaxic surgery dates back to the nineteenth century when its use was pioneered by veterinary surgeons. It was not until the 1930s that the frame was used for surgery on Parkinson's patients. By today's standards, these early procedures were crude, even barbaric. The procedure was little more than trial and error and the results were often less than satisfactory. In one American case reported in 1951, first the motor cortex was disconnected, then other connecting fibres were cut and finally the head of the caudate was severed, which finally relieved the Parkinson's symptoms. It is hard to imagine that there was much brain function left.

Meanwhile, in the 1960s, the potency of L-dopa medications became recognized as far superior to herbal extracts and their synthetic clones, and to some extent replaced surgery as a treatment for Parkinson's. But L-dopa has its limitations. In my case and many others, it produces dyskinesia as a side effect. As these limitations became recognized, stereotaxic surgery was undergoing a revolution in technique resulting from the application of computer technology and miniaturization of surgical instrumentation. Technology assisted as well in understanding the geography of the brain and the specific function of many of the parts of the human brain.

As the two neurosurgeons discussed the operation with me, I realized for the first time how much responsibility for its success would fall on my shoulders. I would have no anaesthetic because there would be no pain. I needed to be alert and mentally clear so I could give timely and accurate responses to the surgeons' questions, particularly about the location of the optic tract, a scant one millimetre from the globus pallidus, and itself only one millimetre in diameter. Should the probe damage the optic tract, my vision could be impaired. If the procedure resulted in bleeding, a stroke could result, with all the complications that come with it, including the possibility of death.

Somehow, all the cautions and potential problems that Dr. Tasker discussed were insignificant when Dr. Lozano described the potential benefits of the operation: moderation of dyskinesia, easing of muscular rigidity on my left side (the operation was going to be on the right side of my brain) and a lessening of the reptilian appearance my Parkinsonian mask had given me. Dr. Lozano had estimated the risk of something going seriously wrong at between 2 and 3 percent. The two surgeons were putting benefits and possible hazards of the operation clearly so that I would be able to sign a "Statement of Informed Consent," a document that says that I understand the risks of the procedure and consent to it being performed.

I realized how desperate my situation was. That videotape at our dinner party had put it to me very graphically. Realistically, I was only months, and at the best a few years, away from having to be put in a chronic care facility. That was enough incentive for me to give the go-ahead. A 97 percent chance that there would be some improvement in my Parkinsonian symptoms seemed to me good odds and I was determined to approach the operation as positively as possible.

Even so, I could not forget the risks involved. During the night before the operation, I was tossing and turning and not sleeping well, my unease increased by being off all my meds. The nurse had been adamant that I would have neither medication nor breakfast. "Doctor's orders," she said. My appeal to Dr. Lozano was rejected out of hand. As I lay awake, I looked out the window of my hospital room and beheld a garish blue neon sign that flashed "Cardinal Funeral Home."

"Is that where they send the ones that don't make it?" I wondered. A variety of images of death, embalming, coffins, and cremation flitted through my mind,

At 7:30 in the morning, Dr. Lozano arrived to take me down to the radiology floor. I sensed that there was still a mixture of wonder and humility hiding behind his shyness, qualities that would not inhibit his single-minded dedication to the tasks of the day whether it was teaching his mentor, Ronald Tasker, the fine points of pallidotomy, or saying during the operation, when I said it might be nice to go to the bathroom, "Tie a string around it." I was definitely on edge with, I hoped, my bravado masking trepidation as I carried on a conversation about leading edge technology with the surgeon.

When we got to the radiology room, I was to have a titanium stereotaxic frame fitted around my head so that an MRI-scan could be done on my brain. To our intense frustration the frame did not fit. "Shit," we said in frustrated unison.

"I have used this frame on over three hundred patients, and you are the first one it hasn't fit," said Lozano.

I explained that I had an unusually large head, size 8 1/4, and that I had always had difficulty getting a hat to fit.

Lozano replied, "I don't think you realize just how serious this is. No frame, no surgery." He then remembered an older steel frame that he thought might be larger.

Back I went to my room while they looked high and low for the older steel frame. It was still early—about 8:15a.m. Determined not to be disappointed by this turn of events, I phoned Tony Graham at the Wellesley, where he is Chief of Cardiology, and asked him to check with their neurosurgeons and find out if they had a frame that would fit. They did not. Now, I really felt dejected. (I was told later that Dr. Lozano was kidded about this by his colleagues: "Andres, do you always send your patients out looking for surgical equipment?")

After an anxious forty-five minute wait, a hospital porter came to take me back to the fitting room. Drs.

Lozano and Tasker were there, waiting. "I found it," said Lozano.

"Let's hope it fits," was my gloomy response.

It did, just.

Dr. Lozano fitted the finely calibrated steel stereotaxic frame around my head and injected local aesthetic at four points where the frame was going to be screwed into my skull. The injection of the anaesthetic was the most painful part of the operation—and it was a pre-operative procedure. When the syringe's needle hit a nerve just above my eyebrow it was excruciating for about a minute. But it made the rest of the fitting and adjusting bearable.

Dr. Tasker reached into a drawer and took out a Black & Decker cordless drill. "They're better and cost a tenth of what the surgical supply houses try to foist on us," he said. In some British hospitals, a stainless steel manual brace and bit is used, supposedly because patients are frightened by the sound of an electric drill.

Dr. Tasker parted the skin and drilled four holes into but not through the bone. The frame was held in place with set screws, which Dr. Lozano tightened against my skull with a crescent wrench. I looked like a blacksmith's idea of Frankenstein's monster.

The downside to using the steel frame was that it could not be used in an MRI-scan; the surgeons would have to make do with images of my brain from the older CAT-scan, which are not of such high quality. I was taken from the examining room on the radiology floor to the CAT-scan room. It took about half an hour to get a set of brain films.

At about 10:45a.m., an orderly wheeled me on a gurney to the operating room, steered it parallel to the operating table, and locked the wheels. I moved myself over to the table. Dr. Lozano bolted the frame surrounding my head to the table, removed a swatch of my hair with barbers' clippers, checked co-ordinates, made a small "x" on my skull with a marking pen and gave it a squirt of local anaesthetic. Dr. Tasker picked up the Black & Decker and drilled a hole three millimetres in diameter through my skull. The only sensation was the acrid bouquet of the bit going through bone.

The low tech, home toolbox part of the day was over.

OR 6 on the second floor of the Toronto Hospital, Toronto Western Division is the neurosurgical room, and it is filled with computers that do everything from recording individual brain cell activity to mapping the geography of the brain. Dr. Tasker assured me, the Black & Decker notwithstanding, that only the very latest equipment and instruments were being used. "We could not have performed these procedures with anything like the precision and accuracy we do now as recently as two years ago," he said.

As they began literally probing into my brain on their way to the globus pallidus, the surgeons were in effect working blind. They could not see my brain cells and the navigation was done by a neurophysiologist with a detailed, computerized knowledge of the brain's geography who relied on the "noise" the cells produced when touched by a probe. The probes are very fine, small instruments, about six inches long and two millimetres in diameter, capable of probing individual brain cells and accepting data from them. Without the information generated by the probe, the OR team would be like a child's birthday party playing Pin the Tail on the Donkey.

For a patient, a pallidotomy is a long, sometimes tedious, but demanding and exciting operation. It was a real adventure—being wide awake while they were fixing my brain. During the first four hours, five cross-sections of the globus pallidus, each 15mm square, were probed, cell by individual cell. Each time the surgeons probed a different cell, they asked me either to stick out my tongue (a small child's delight, but for an adult—me—the novelty wore off pretty quickly), clench and unclench my left hand, or make a kicking motion with my left leg. Sometimes, one of the staff would move the leg or arm to see if passive activity had a different effect on cell response than active movement. It seemed odd—and marvelous—that the neurosurgeons could pinpoint brain cells within a cross-section and predict, based on surgical experience, what specific part of the body that cell controlled.

The information generated by the cell probe and muscle movements were all stored in a computer for current use and future study. The Western Hospital has developed a proprietary software programme that generates extremely precise three dimensional images of each of the sections of the brain being examined. All the data was input before deciding the location of the lesions, the single critical decision in the whole operating procedure. As well, the surgeons stimulated cells to determine the location of the optic tract. When the tract was stimulated, I saw cascading pins of light.

The surgeons consulted the neurophysiologist, who had been doing the brain mapping about the optimal size and location of the lesions. The data generated two images: one of my brain and one of the average of my brain and the brains of the thirteen other people who had had pallidotomies before me. Using all this information, the surgeons and the neurophysiologist decided on the location of the lesions.

The decisive moment was approaching. A probe was heated to 90° Celsius to make the lesions. In this procedure, the lesions were made by a heated probe, which is capable of more precise and accurate lesioning than a scalpel. (Cryosurgery—using a frozen probe that creates lesions by freezing the tissue—is another technique. The neurosurgeons believed the instrumentation for that technique was clumsier.)

As Dr. Tasker positioned the probe at the precise location in my brain and then heated the probe, making the lesions, I felt the rigidity leaving my left side. It was an eerie, supernatural experience and it only took ninety seconds.

Dr. Lozano asked me to pretend that I was putting a light bulb in its socket with my left hand. This is a common clinical test used to observe the degree of slowness and clumsiness in a Parkinson's patient. Watching me, Jan Duff, who had conducted the pre-op tests, said with triumph in her voice, "That is better than his best 'on.'"

The surgeons had transformed my life.

I moved myself back to the gurney to go back to my room, and shook hands with the surgical team (how often can you do that right in the operating room?). I was wheeled back to my hospital room where Esther, Howard, and Stephen Booth were waiting anxiously. The telephone rang. "Its probably for me," I said jumping from the gurney and walking quickly to the phone. It was Emily, wanting to know how the operation had gone.

"What's all the commotion?" she asked. I told her it was just the hospital staff clucking about like mother hens: patients are not supposed to jump off gurneys to answer phones on the way back from major brain surgery.

That evening, in a bout of post-operative euphoria, I decided to walk down to the lobby and get a Coke and a pizza. I only made half the round trip. My legs buckled as I started back from the hospital's pizza place. It was nothing more or less than utter physical exhaustion. No harm was done.

The very day of my operation, 1,080 copies of my book A Transforming Influence, a biographical memoir of Archbishop Howard H. Clark were delivered to our house. I felt this was more than coincidence; it was Providential. I gave autographed copies with the inscription "with thanks for transforming my life" to each of Dr. Lang, Dr. Lozano, Dr. Tasker, and Jan Duff.

Dr. Tasker and Dr. Lozano had worked a miracle on me. My left side was no longer rigid, and when I was on meds, I had no left side dyskinesia. It worked normally. Even though I had been fully involved in the whole operation I found it hard to understand how making lesions on such a small part of my brain could have such a profound effect.

The recovery time from the operation was very short. I was home two days later on Friday and on Saturday evening went out to a large party for David Warren's Idler magazine. Before the operation I would have hesitated to go to such a party and Esther would have tried to persuade me not to go—she was more aware than I of the difficulty people had in dealing with me and of the effect of my dyskinesia. David Warren and his people at the magazine had put up with me through the worst of my Parkinson's and I was warmly greeted the staff of the magazine who all could see the change in me more than I could. Everyone noticed the absence of dyskinesia. I realized people were much easier with me socially, and they no longer had to give me a wide birth to avoid the hazard of dyskinesia.

It all seemed too simple to have such a profound effect.

Here is the end of my poem, "Lazarus."

V

Waiting. Endlessly...
Preparation, three days of tests
Word games, memory, spatial,
Meds on ... meds off ... performance
Videotaping me walking, moving and immobile
The Social Contract, so-called...
Richard Hooker looks down in horror
The perverted use of noble thought
Destroys the polity.
Hence the waiting
For an O.R.
False alarms ... then
Go back home.

VI

Skull bolted to the table
Immobilized
For the duration.
Wide awake. No Sedation.

The only sensation
The acrid bouquet
Of the drill going through bone.

Thee hundred minutes in the O.R.
Alert.
It worked.
An end to deformed harmony.

Technology and Humanity
Combine to perform a miracle
There is wonder in life
In God's creation

How do I thank the medical team
They did their jobs
Professionally
Gave me new life.
resurrection

Good cheer and labour on some more
Reap the joy I radiate.
Walking
Laughing.
Your care released me from that older trap.

I am Lazarus.

CHAPTER NINE

A Special Kind of Support

I was euphoric during the first few weeks after the operation, but I gradually realized that only the right side of my body had been effected. This was to be expected since it was the left side of my brain that had been treated. The right side of my body, particularly my leg, was still very much subject to my medications going off, sometimes in the most unpredictable ways.

In spite of this daily handicap, I wanted to enjoy the freedom the operation had given me and I didn't mind taking risks doing it. There were times, glorious times, through the winter and spring of 1994, when my meds were working as they should. I went cross-country skiing for the first time in several years. For my first ski excursion we went to a fairly remote area. If my meds had gone off unexpectedly I would have been stuck there and we would have had real difficulty getting me back to the car, and if they had gone off as I was running downhill I could have hurt myself badly. But these were chances I was prepared to take.

The following summer, I played tennis for the first time in five years, wearing out one of Esther's nieces and her husband with my enthusiasm, if not my skill.

Again, if my meds had gone off when I was in mid-run for a ball I could have had a bad accident, but it didn't happen.

That same summer I delivered two sermons at our church, Christ Church, Deer Park. Perhaps, for some people, this brought to mind Samuel Johnson's no longer politically correct comment concluding "...It is not done well, but you are surprised to find it done at all." I was surprised that I could do it, but delighted as well.

In the months following my operation I began taking an increasingly active part in the Parkinson's Foundation. When I had first been diagnosed with Parkinson's back in 1982, I had responded to the condition with denial and fatalism, and had avoided the Foundation with its do-gooding reputation. Esther had taken a more positive approach, become involved, and used the excellent information service to educate herself about Parkinson's, and she had supported the Foundation in some of its fundraising activities.

The Parkinson Foundation of Canada is the principal organization in Canada representing the interests of people with Parkinson's. Together with affiliated organizations in British Columbia, Alberta, and the National Capital Region, it is a national network. The Foundation's head office is in Toronto. The requirements for local chapters are served by regional offices in St. John's for Newfoundland and Labrador, Halifax for the Maritime provinces, Montreal for

Quebec, Toronto for Central Ontario, and London for Southwestern Ontario.

The Central Ontario Region is the administrative arm of the Foundation serving the Toronto Chapter, the largest and most active in the Foundation. Under the leadership of an executive director, staff services are provided to the chapters and support groups.

My own first connection with the Foundation had ended in disappointment—the cookbook I had written in 1988, which I believed could be a useful fundraiser for the Foundation, had been declined—and, in effect, I went away mad. I stayed away until the winter of 1991-92 when Esther worked on a fundraising event. I helped her, and began to see the value, even the fun, of it. The Toronto Chapter of the Foundation had a newsletter. I thought that with my experience writing for Seven Days magazine I had something to offer, and in the spring of 1992 I joined the executive committee of the Toronto Chapter and became editor of the newsletter.

That I knew little about the Chapter and less about the Foundation did not deter me; it probably made me keener! I didn't just edit the newsletter. I changed its name, wrote most of the articles, and what I didn't write, rewrote. I was sure my style and presentation were better than anyone else's. I edited the newsletter as though I were running my own Time magazine. The Chapter president and the former editor checked my first issue for accuracy, but they did not realize the extent of my editorial activities.

When the newsletter appeared, I felt pleased with my efforts, but it produced a major crisis. I had failed to grasp that the newsletter was a co-operative effort, and that, like other aspects of volunteer work for the Foundation, the hard work of other volunteers had to be acknowledged and respected.

The executive director of the Foundation called me into her office and gave me a terrible dressing down. It was so devastating that I shook for the rest of the day—a Parkinsonian reaction to stress. What she said was correct, but she was ruthless. Subsequently, there was a special meeting of the Chapter executive at which an editorial committee was struck to review each issue prior to publication. That constraint was more than my pride would allow and I decided to resign. It was probably just as well, for I had more than enough to think about. Esther had just been diagnosed with multiple sclerosis, I wanted to complete my biography of Howard Clark, and the major renovation of our house was about to begin. Joan Prior, the new Chapter president, accepted my resignation and graciously said that I would be welcome back on the executive any time.

We had undertaken the renovation of our house so that Esther, with MS, and I, with Parkinson's, could continue to live there comfortably and safely. In April 1993, when the renovation was nearly finished, Esther and I and John Vanstone, our architect, gave a presentation of the renovation at a meeting of the Toronto Chapter of the Parkinson's Foundation. I was making the presentation, but about two sentences in, my speech became slurred and indistinct, so I turned the program over to Esther and John. Much to my surprise, I felt no embarrassment or humiliation; it was just part of having Parkinson's. Despite my poor performance, the evening had gone well, and I felt good about it.

The exciting part of it all was the warmth and open way I was accepted by everyone connected with the Chapter—from the newest member to the founding members who were still active. It took me a while to realize that I was among peers, and that my dyskinesia did not frighten them. Their unquestioning acceptance of me was a kind of peer support I had been missing because of my denial and arrogance.

I also realized that I had been fortunate in a way that many Parkinsonians were not. My friends had been my personal support group. I hadn't gone to them and said, "will you help me cope with Parkinson's by being my support group?" They had just done it: Stephen Booth, Ian Hamilton, Howard Shill, Tony Graham, and a number of others. Through the foundation, I began to realize that there are many Parkinsonians who do not have a supportive family or group of friends to help them through the rough periods.

That spring and summer of 1993, when Parkinson's seemed to be accelerating through my body, I was almost manic in my need for activity and accomplishment. Esther, as part of her work with the Board of Education, had been involved in a group working with inner city children and their behaviour problems. One thing that fascinated me was the health problems that seemed to be endemic there. The data was irrefutable, and led me to try to square my traditional conservative political views with the obvious need for social assistance and social justice.

I was very much influenced by Gertrude Himmelfarb's book Poverty and Compassion: the moral imagination of the late Victorians. She describes how the Victorians transformed their passion for religion into compassion for humanity. But most people in nineteenth-century Britain and North America shared the common ideology of Christianity. This is no longer the case in late twentieth-century Canada. I wanted to find a system of nationally shared values that might, on the surface, be similar to what we call our Judaeo- Christian heritage, but it would differ in the richness of nuance and subtlety that comes from its being forged in the crucible of national debate. It would surely affirm the dignity of human life and the concept of humanity being a product of God's imagination. I recognized that such a concept already existed in Toronto, with programmes such as "Out of the Cold," in which seven churches (one for each day of the week) provided a hot dinner, bed, and breakfast for the homeless on an ideology-free basis.

The philosophical problem I saw was that as long as these services were provided without thought of compensation by the state, the institutions providing them earned the right to speak for those they served; if they sought compensation, they would be simply another contractor in the social assistance system. In addition, I began to understand that the group served could only be represented by the sponsoring institutions in the short term. As the group served became cohesive, its members needed to learn the art of self-advocacy. This process might be painful for the originating sponsors as they might find themselves attacked or seeing points of view espoused that seemed contrary to the originating values.

During the summer, the more I thought about it, the more I became concerned about this issue. I talked about it at length at Blue Sea with Tony Graham, and back in Toronto with Stephen Booth and Tony Lang. I wrote a paper that I wanted to present to the Toronto Chapter of the Parkinson Foundation. I showed Joan Prior a draft. Although my proposal was clearly not part of her agenda, she recognized it as a legitimate viewpoint and invited me to present it at the September meeting of the Chapter. She also invited me again to rejoin the executive of the Toronto Chapter.

The paper, titled Does Toronto Have a Soul?: a challenge to the Toronto chapter of the Parkinson foundation of Canada, argued that, despite Canada's universal health insurance, there were a lot of people with undiagnosed Parkinson's and other chronic diseases living in Toronto's inner city as a result of society's sin of omission: not providing sufficient health care resources to deliver the same standard of care to the homeless and indigent as is available to rest of society. Society, I argued, had—and has—a positive obligation to remedy this failure. The task was daunting: to do it properly would involve a colossal unified effort of business, labour, the city, and the provincial and federal governments to eliminate the factors leading to poor health in the inner city. But that was no reason to not make a start.

The proposal was well-received when I presented it at the September meeting. However, I soon realized that I could not expect the Chapter to drop everything and re-orient itself to my agenda. As Matthew Arnold said, "it is not a having and getting, but a growing and becoming."

At that same meeting, Joan asked for volunteers for the position of vice-president, with the plan being to succeed her in six months time. After thinking about it for a few weeks, I called Joan and asked her if she would accept me in that position. She responded positively and through October and November I began to immerse myself in the Chapter's affairs. I soon found that I had a good deal to learn—from the exercise groups and Taoist Tai Chi classes to the various support groups co-ordinated by the Chapter as well as the all-important question of fundraising.

During this time I was also winding up for my pallidotomy operation, which took place in December. Because the operation was so successful and I recovered from it so quickly, I was able to maintain my momentum in the Chapter activities. One day, a few weeks after the operation, I was at the hospital for a routine follow-up appointment when Jan Duff asked me if I would see a patient who was going to have a pallidotomy the next day. It was Peter Kingston, a former president of the Toronto Chapter of the Parkinson's Foundation. He was quite apprehensive about the operation, and we talked for about an hour. I told him about my experience and about the anxieties I had had. When I left, he was looking forward to the operation. I stopped in on Peter the day after his operation. The change was so great in him and was so positive that I was moved to tears.

I began to see other prospective patients and these visits developed into one of the Central Ontario Region's initiatives, the Peer Support Programme, in which Parkinsonian's, particularly those of us who have had surgical or other special treatment provide advice and encouragement to others. I have now seen or spoken to over a hundred Parkinson's patients who were considering surgery to alleviate their symptoms and it gives me great satisfaction.

Of course the conversation varies with every patient, but centres on the Parkinsonian experience, what it has meant to the patient and to me. Typical questions are: is the operation painful? how does it feel emotionally when the lesions are made? what is my confidence level with the surgeons? how long does it take? is all the neuropsychological testing necessary? how much improvement should be expected? In discussing these subjects I have had to be careful that I offer no medical opinion and am not critical of any doctors. And, of course, I have to be careful in talking about what the operation has done for me. I have to be candid and say that there are no guarantees; these procedures do not come with an owner's manual. I always stress that my results, which are the best the surgical team has achieved to date, may not be replicated.

Most of the operations are successful and I am almost always emotional when I see the pleasure and excitement of the patient. I have become almost a fixture at the hospital, so much so that occasionally I have taken certain liberties. Dr. Andres Lozano said to me recently, his tongue only half in his cheek: "Bill, this is a hospital. As a general rule, the doctors make rounds on the patients, not the other way round. I fully expect to hear on the public address system an announcement that "Mr. Harshaw will be conducting pallidotomy rounds at 2p.m."

After my December 1993 operation, I became even more active in the Chapter and Foundation. I became president of the Toronto Chapter at its Annual Meeting in April 1994 and in September I was nominated to the board of the Foundation.

I gradually saw that the kind of support the Chapter and the Foundation were giving me was unique, as is the support they gave everyone. For me, that support was the unquestioning acceptance of me as a person with Parkinson's and the willingness to listen and consider my ideas. That might not sound like a great deal of support, but it was vital to me.

Back in the days when I worked at Molson's, I had enjoyed a high level of responsibility. I had been unable to replicate this when I worked at the bank. Intellectually, I could accept that this was an inevitable consequence of my Parkinson's, but it still bothered me. Now, at the Foundation, I felt back on track. I was involved in a cause I felt committed to and where my business experience could be put to work. Initially, Esther had to restrain me. I was out to recreate the world in six days, and never mind resting on the seventh day. As I reined myself in, I reached back to Molson days and remembered some of the lessons I had learned there from mentors like Jim Black and Drew McCaughey such as the importance of sharing the credit and taking the blame. And vision. It is essential to have a clear idea of the goals and objectives you want an organization to strive for. Initially I did not know what my vision for the Foundation was.

As it evolved, it was simple. I wanted the Chapter, and then the Foundation, to develop into more accountable bodies, working for the stakeholders, above all for Parkinsonians, and answerable to them. Until this time the Foundation and the Chapter had been in the first stage of a service and advocacy body—the governance was almost entirely in the hands of the executive, which was essentially self-appointing. I believed the time had come to extend the governance to the membership at large by expanding the nomination committee and inviting nominations from the membership, and having the directors properly elected by the members. Likewise, by moving the Annual General Meeting until later in the year, when the Chapter's annual financial statements were ready, these could be properly approved by the membership. It was also time to recognize the professional nature of the Toronto staff and to formalize and write job descriptions of the various positions.

I came to realize that the volunteers are the most important people in the Foundation. Staff co-ordinate and provide administrative services, but without volunteers, there is no Foundation. They never let us forget that we exist to serve Parkinsonians and their community. The volunteers are the grass roots we dare not lose touch with.

I soon discovered that all my waking hours could be spent on Chapter business. I had to resist this. There were some events that I had to attend, but there were not that many of them. Leadership means trusting those in positions of responsibility to do the job. Despite my enthusiasm, I realized that I should not appear at all the committee meetings or I would give the impression that I had little confidence in the committee chair. And, I recognized, I am not a good detail person, and often the committees spend a lot of time on details, as they must.

In the next years we made some strong advances in fund raising, in particular with our annual tulip sale and in the SuperWalk for Parkinson's. Charity walks had become a bit commonplace and we had to find ways to set this one apart. In 1993 the walk raised only $14,000. As Chapter president I had to support the event and by using all my contacts was able to raise $3000 out of a total of $20,000.

But one person should not be raising 15 percent of the revenue. The 1995 Walk had a number of new features: a new logo and theme slogan "We walk to help those who have difficulty walking," international participation and a tripling of gross funds raised to over $60,000. I sent out sixty-nine letters and raised $4,300. The difference was that in 1995, I was in fourth place in sponsorship pledges.

For the 1996 SuperWalk, the Toronto project that had started small had grown to twenty-three cities in Canada, the United States, and several European countries. As well, the Foundation has secured Major-General Lewis MacKenzie as National Honourary

Chairman and the Honourable David Crombie as Honourary Toronto Chairman. The volunteer team has done a superb job in growing SuperWalk from being a local event to being a major, international fundraising event.

The continuing challenge for all the chapters of the Foundation is to reach all those Parkinsonians and families who could benefit from the support of the Foundation. At present the Toronto Chapter has about five hundred members, just over 6 percent of the estimated number of Parkinsonians in the Greater Toronto Area. This is slightly below the national average 9 percent. I worry about whether we can be an effective advocate with such a low share of the market. We have to become more effective in marketing the advantages of membership to Parkinsonians and their caregivers. It is sad and sometimes tragic that such a large proportion of people with Parkinson's suffers in silence and loneliness.

One of our 1994 initiatives was spectacularly successful and extended well beyond Parkinson's. The cost of medications is a major social problem that, ironically, becomes more serious with each major discovery by the pharmaceutical industry. As the technology for discovery becomes more expensive, so do the drugs. Consequently, without a good drug insurance programme or government assistance programme, the financial implications of chronic illnesses to individuals and families can be catastrophic.

In Ontario at this time, the Drug Benefit Plan, one of the cornerstones of the Provincial Health Plan, was essentially a list, known as the Formulary, of drugs that could be provided free of charge to seniors and to people on social assistance. Although the Ontario Drug Benefit Plan, as it existed, did provide coverage for a wide range of medicines, it did not provide secure coverage for people who had chronic diseases, and it gave no help to people of limited means. Poorer families were having to go on social assistance in order to be funded for the necessary medications for long-term diseases and medical conditions—everything from AIDS to renal failure. And they were losing their dignity in the process. The inequity was tremendous, because the cost of drug therapy varied so much for different conditions. For some medical conditions, the cost of regular drugs was crippling even for people in the highest tax bracket.

For Parkinsonian's, the important medications are controlled release (CR) and sustained release (SR) drugs, some of which were on the formulary. One of them, Sinemet CR (which I used) was not on the formulary as it was a fairly new adaption of an existing drug. Seniors and those on welfare could get Sinemet CR for free, but only after having obtained special permission from the Ministry of Health. This was routinely granted, but only after a lengthy and frustrating process. At a meeting of the Foundation board, we heard that the Ministry of Health was now considering removing controlled release and sustained release medications altogether. Some had already been taken off the list on the grounds that they were inefficacious. Frank Roth, the bubbling, witty entertainment lawyer who was president of the Foundation, had read my "Does Toronto Have a Soul" speech. He came to me and in his comical, mock "Man from Uncle" voice said "Your assignment, should you accept, is to devise a drug plan which will cover all Parkinsonians."

I accepted with alacrity and with no realization of what a huge task it was. In approaching the problem, we had to recognize that, with the province's huge financial deficit, the Minister of Health had the unenviable task of having to bake a smaller pie and then carve it up among the ministry's many supplicants. For the first time the health budget was being reduced. It was also obvious that the problem of drug costs was not just limited to Parkinsonians.

Our goal was to devise a practical proposal for a drug plan for chronic illnesses that we could put to the government. It was ambitious, but the need was great. We had to do more than bewail the problem. We knew that it was unrealistic as well as perhaps undesirable to demand free access to all drugs on demand. We were looking for a formula that combined private co-payment with government funding.

We involved the Toronto Chapter's very capable executive director Maggie Wheelock and the whole executive committee. Most importantly, in order to make sure we stayed on the rails and came up with a practical proposal we could put to the government, we established a review committee made up of tax, medical, and health care experts. It included Dr. Anthony Graham, Chief of Cardiology, The Wellesley Hospital; Dr. Anthony Lang, Director, Movement Disorders, The Toronto Hospital; Robert Lindsay, Senior Tax Partner, Osler Hoskin Harcourt; Thomas McDonnell, Executive Director, The Canadian Tax Foundation; and Trevor Williams, then the Chief Executive Officer, The Parkinson Foundaton of Canada. The key member of the committee was Michael Decter, former Deputy Minister of Health for Ontario. The review committee was essential in ensuring the practicality of our proposal: many of its suggestions were incorporated in the final document.

We had to face an important issue at a meeting of the review committee in September. The AIDS Committee of Toronto was the only other group that had seriously addressed the issue of long-term drug costs. We had invited representatives of the AIDS Committee to join although we knew that they were philosophically opposed to the notion of co-payment. The AIDS representatives were of the view that everyone has a right of access to needed medications free of charge. We clashed at the meeting, but it was a polite disagreement.

The challenge was to devise a plan that is universal, i.e. available as a right to all residents of Ontario, while at the same time being progressive, i.e. the private co-payment would increase relative to the individual's income. After many drafts we arrived at a plan that satisfied the review committee. Here is a simplified example of the proposal:

Net income, family of 3:	$20,000	$40,000	$60,000
Annual prescription cost:	$5,000	$5,000	$5,000
Prescription cost as % of income:	25%	12.5%	8.3%
Proposed co-payment:	$350	$1,239	$2,139
Co-payment as % of income:	1.8%	3.1%	3.6%

We decided to present it at the annual meeting of the Foundation in Montreal in September, 1994. I made the presentation with the title "Restoring Dignity."

After I finished, I was walked back to my seat and wondered why people were standing up. Frank Roth, the president, said "Bill, they are giving you a standing ovation. This has never happened before."

Why the standing ovation? Our presentation gave Parkinsonians hope—hope that the Foundation was looking out for their interests. I then moved, seconded by David Black, a past president, that my speech become Foundation policy.

A day later, through Michael Decter's good offices, I was invited to participate in a consultation meeting to consider our proposal. The meeting was sponsored by the National Pharmaceutical Strategy Directorate of Health Canada. It was a great success, but we were not optimistic about its chances of being adopted by the Ontario government in the near term.

To the astonishment of most of us, only a couple of months later, on December 1, 1994, the Premier of Ontario, Bob Rae, announced the government's Trillium Drug Plan, which was modeled in all important respects on "Restoring Dignity."

At a press conference in Toronto, the Minister of Health, Ruth Grier, announced the plan in detail, including the size of the co-payment. I was invited to make a statement at the conference. After the questions were over, Mrs. Grier publicly thanked me for the impact I had on the plan's design, and joked, "it's not very often that a lifelong Tory like you is the author of an NDP program."

The Trillium Drug Programme as introduced by Premier Rae's NDP government still had a problem in that the deductible structure or the co-payment provisions were not progressive enough. There were only three break points at which the level of co-payment changed and these kicked in at lower rather than higher incomes.

We urged the new Conservative government of Mike Harris to make the plan more equitable so that the primary beneficiaries will be those with low incomes by using break points which would result in lower co-payments for low income levels and higher copayments for those with higher incomes. These recommendations were accepted by the government.

Our experience with the Trillium Drug Plan really began the Chapter and Foundation leadership in advocacy matters on issues that concern all Parkinsonians. The process taught us a valuable lesson. In dealing with government, the approach should not be prescriptive, telling the government in no uncertain terms what to do. You are more likely to get a favourable hearing and to be successful if your proposal is descriptive of the problem, offering alternative solutions, allowing the government to take its own initiative.

For me, the experience of working on the Trillium plan and other Foundation activities has been a tremendous opportunity. I have become virtually a professional Parkinsonian, putting my experience of my years with Parkinson's in combination with my business skills. My goal in this work is to make the Parkinsonian experience easier for those who will come after. It has been part of the process of learning and of intellectual and spiritual freedom that I have called my adventure with Parkinson's.

CHAPTER TEN

Doing the Other Side

The announcement of the Trillium Drug Plan at the beginning of December 1994 was a tremendous victory for people in Ontario with chronic diseases and it was an important step forward for the Parkinson's Foundation and for the Toronto Chapter. It was also important for me in a personal way because it validated the work I had done on the project and gave me a new level of confidence. At this time I needed to feel as positive and enthusiastic as possible because I was, just ten days after the Trillium announcement, going to have a second operation on my brain, one that was going to be a medical first for the neurosurgical team and which would need all the reserves of confidence and stamina I could muster.

The pallidotomy I had had a year before had been wonderfully successful as far as it went and I had the experience and exhilaration of enjoying again activities like walking, fly fishing, skiing, going shopping, and the normal activities of daily life, as well as a much greater ease in social life and communication. But the operation had only affected one side of my body and, in the months after my operation, Parkinson's did not stand still. As a result, there was a paradox in my condition.

While I retained the benefits of the operation on my left side, movement rigidity was an increasing problem on my right side. Despite the fact that I could sometimes ski and play tennis, I also could not walk unaided for as much as five hours a day when my meds were off. I found an account by Oliver Sacks, talking about another situation, that described my feelings well:

> The leg was in exile ... or it was not where it should be. Normally we are so at home in our bodies and we so own them that things like this are unimaginable.

Despite the satisfaction from the work I was doing with the Parkinson Foundation and the pleasure of being more active again, the restrictions Parkinson's made on me were sometimes overwhelmingly oppressive. One day in November I went to see a friend, John Fraser, a well-known journalist and Toronto personality who had an office at Massey College at the University of Toronto. After checking in at the Porter's Lodge, I started to cross the quadrangle to John's staircase. Only I didn't. After a few steps, I froze. My meds went off. My normal stride of eighty centimetres had shrunk to little more than one centimetre. I was crawling on my feet. Christ, it was going to take forever to get there, only about a hundred metres. People noticed me—it was hard not to. Luckily I had my cane with me so I didn't go tumbling to the ground. Thank God! A few asked if they could help. Stupidly, I said, "Oh, no I'm alright. Its just my Parkinson's acting up."

John saw me from his window and came rushing to my side. "Bill, this is terrible. I had no idea Parkinson's affected you so much. How can I help? We'll go to the Common Room, its not as far as my rooms."

With John's support we made halting progress until we reached the stairs. These I could manage and I bounded up with alacrity, only to resume my snail's crawl when we reached the landing.

I was beginning to think about writing a book about my experience with Parkinson's and wanted to talk to him about it. As we chatted, John put me totally at ease, and for one of the few times, I recounted my private agony of Parkinson's, how I feared feeling freak-like and unwanted. It was hard, because I didn't want to feel sorry for myself, nor did I want others to feel sorry for me. I was terrified that my Parkinson's would land me in a chronic care hospital utterly immobilized and incapacitated: that's why I increasingly felt like Francis Bacon's screaming pope, disenfranchised and disempowered. John encouraged me to talk about this and eventually said, "Bill, people accept you for what you are not what you have. Only the ignorant and the insecure don't accept your disability. Ignore them."

I felt as though I had been to confession, because it was rare for me to unburden my soul. John gave me a copy of his new book Saturday Night Lives and inscribed it "To William Harshaw, with respect."

When I left an hour later, my meds were back on and I was refreshed and rejuvenated by John's understanding and compassion.

It had been clear soon after the first operation that if I was to have the benefit of increased mobility in a dependable way, something would have to be done to my right side. The need to be able to help Esther was the main reason for my having been chosen for surgery in the first place, but I was of little use to her with my right side going off without warning. Dr. Lang soon came to the conclusion we should take the next step. In April 1994, only four months after my operation, he said, "The other side must be done. It's risky, because we will be in uncharted territory, but the risk is outweighed by the benefits."

I had many conversations with him over the course of the next eight months, most of them late at night when he had time to talk at length. He went into considerable detail, reporting findings as he heard of them.

There were really two alternatives for the surgeons, other than to do nothing: either a second unilateral pallidotomy, which would make it bilateral, or chronic deep brain stimulation, a rather more sensational procedure.

No bilateral pallidotomies had been performed in Canada, but there were some data from foreign surgical centres indicating that a bilateral pallidotomy could produce serious complications such as cognitive, speech, and gait problems. Hence there was a reluctance to perform this operation. (The Toronto neurosurgeons have subsequently done two bilaterals, one with serious complications.)

Chronic deep brain stimulation, the second possibility, produces the same effect as a pallidotomy by a different method. In a pallidotomy, brain cells are lesioned—in fact destroyed—in order to normalize the brain's electrical activity. In chronic deep brain stimulation, two electrodes are implanted in the brain, one in the globus pallidus (GPI) and the other in the sub-thalamic nucleus (STN), part of the basal ganglia. The electrodes are connected to a neurostimulator, which is similar to the cardiac pacemaker that many heart patients use. It produces a constant tiny electrical charge that normalizes electrical activity in the two brain areas where, before, Parkinson's disease had caused irregular transmissions and receptions. One advantage of chronic deep brain stimulation compared to a pallidotomy is that there is the possibility of reversing it—the electrodes could be withdrawn if the stimulation produces an unwanted condition.

This was the procedure chosen by Dr. Lozano and his colleagues. I was made very much a part of the decision process because this would be the first time in North America that chronic stimulation would be attempted in the basal ganglia. Less than half-a-dozen cases were on record, performed in Grenoble, France.

At the beginning of December, a couple of weeks before the operation was scheduled, I went in for another round of pre-operative neuro-psychological tests. They were the same tests that I had taken the previous year, which I thought might compromise the test outcome. In the event, I did not remember enough from the first round of testing, or from my post-operative assessment, to make any difference.

The operation was scheduled for Wednesday, December 14. I was admitted to hospital the day before. After I was settled in, Dr. Lozano saw me in his office for about an hour. "I know you have discussed this with Dr. Lang," he began, "but I must be sure that you understand not only the potential benefits but also the risks of deep brain stimulation." He went on to say that, while the final decision would not be made until during the operation when they were in my brain, their thinking was that DBS was the procedure of choice.

Apart from the actual procedure being performed, there would be a number of "firsts" connected with the operation, the most significant of which was the first recording of cell activity in a human sub-thalamic nucleus. Quite apart from being an interesting addition to scientific knowledge, it underscores the Western Hospital's approach to research surgery: it must have an empirical basis as well as a theoretical foundation. Inference from laboratory animals and from theory is not good enough. There must be observable evidence. While this is a more conservative approach, it is safer and reduces surgical risk.

I knew more about the second operation than the first, about the risks and potential benefits. I tried to ignore the risks, real though they were, and simply put myself in Lozano's and Tasker's hands. I did this because the risks were too horrible to contemplate: cognitive deterioration, balance and gait problems and further speech problems. Simply put, I had a faith in my two neurosurgeons' abilities that overrode any potential problems.

Much of the operation would be similar to the one I had had a year before. Using the stereotaxic frame and drilling holes into my skull, they would probe into the globus pallidus area of my brain and record brain cell activity by cross-section, the surgeons working with great precision and to close tolerances. Again, I would be awake and must be alert during the entire procedure.

However, this time, there would be more cross-sections of my brain examined and then there would be the insertion of the electrodes; I should expect surgical trauma and edema. There would be extensive testing required after the operation, and again some days or weeks later, before the pacemaker would be attached to activate the electrodes. Mostly

I was excited by the prospect of the second operation, because of the possibility of further alleviation of my symptoms and also because I was going to be a medical pioneer. Esther was more apprehensive than I was because of the unknown factor. One of her aphorisms was "the patient has the operation; the family lives with the consequences." Howard and Emily were both apprehensive and excited—they were fearful of a screw-up but were excited by the possibility my having my mobility restored. They were both still teenagers, and however loyal and loving they were, they must have suffered terrible embarrassment from having a father with such a disconcerting and strange condition.

That night as I lay in the hospital waiting for the operation the next morning, I was excited but not relaxed. In fact, I was really on edge. I tossed and turned and did not sleep well at all. I knew the next day's operation was going to be even longer and more demanding than the last one, and that I needed to be well rested but sleep would not come. About 3:30 in the morning I turned the light on and read for a while, but I don't think I absorbed much. As morning came, I heard the hospital gradually waking up, tired residents and interns and nurses going off their shift, greeting grumpy, half-awake colleagues coming in trying to be civil. I was ravenously hungry, but was not allowed to have any breakfast, and I was pretty well immobile because I was off my medications.

I was prepared for this operation to be longer and more complex and demanding than my first operation, though it would replicate much of it. First there was the fitting of the stereotaxic frame on my head. Again they used the old steel frame, because with the size of my head I again could not use the newer titanium frame. The OR staff were used to the newer frame and had to remind themselves of the eccentricities of the older one. It was old hat to me, so to speak, or so I thought. I had repressed the memory of the single painful part of the first operation—the injection of local anaesthetic into a nerve just above my eyebrow. It was excruciating, but lasted only a minute. Then followed the CAT-scan, the wait in the surgical waiting room and finally I was rolled into the operating room.[7]

In addition to Dr. Tasker and Dr. Lozano, there was a third neurosurgeon in this procedure, Dr. Michael Munz, a Neurosurgical Fellow working here under the supervision of Dr. Tasker and Dr. Lozano to learn more about the sub-specialty—stereotaxic surgery and functional neurosurgery. From his qualification as a surgeon, Munz had been studying for ten years, meaning thirteen years after his medical degree. He masked his professional concentration by seeming to be pretty blasé about the whole affair, treating it as just another day's work. I was quite cross with him because he was pricking my balloon of excitement and enthusiasm and deflating me. I knew we were all in for a long hard day and decided that it would be a good idea to start the morning off with a joke. When the stereotaxic frame was on and Michael Munz was removing some hair from my head, I said, "It's a good thing you aren't trying to make a living as a hair stylist, Munz, you'd go bankrupt, unless you're trying to be a Sweeney Todd."

"Who is Sweeney Todd?", he replied.

"Munz, are you a complete illiterate? Those were the days when barbers doubled as surgeons—or was it surgeons doubling as barbers? Don't they teach you anything about the history of medicine here?"

My joke fell flat. Munz became awfully quiet. Someone observed: "Michael's really pissed off."

I really had been pretty tactless, suggesting to a professional of Munz's calibre that he was illiterate. He just didn't know of the Broadway musical of the late 1970s, Sweeney Todd, the Demon Barber of Fleet Street.

Dr. Lozano broke the ice by saying: "Dr. Munz, Mr. Harshaw makes even neurosurgeons laugh at themselves."

He and Dr. Tasker were ready with the Black & Decker drill and soon I could smell the acrid bouquet of the drill going through my skull. Then the operation became dull and tedious for me as they probed through my brain, recording its activity cell by cell, asking me what I felt or perceived.

Dr. Munz had created a computer programme that mapped the brain. This was a different "map" than the one used in the first operation because the left Globus Pallidus was being investigated rather than the right and the sub-thalamic nucleus had never been mapped before. This programme could be used to aggregate the data for patients in a study group, and show how the current patient differed from the average. Work such as this enables Lozano's and Tasker's research surgery to be performed with lower risk than would otherwise be the case.

About mid-way through the thirteen cross sections, we were in uncharted territory, making the first recording in medical history of cell activity in the sub-thalamic nucleus, one of the target areas for electrode placement. Because this area of the brain had never had cell activity recorded, there were not be any tell-tale noises from the computer to help our brain mapper know exactly where we were.

Excitement gave way to tedium and then to boredom, a bit like sailing for a long time with a constant wind on one tack with perfectly trimmed sails. But there was always a sense of adventure lingering because the surgeons were exploring where no one had been before. Also, as the recordings of cell activity were made with the insertion of electrodes in mind rather than lesioning, the perspective was altered. The globus pallidus was approached from a different plane.

Implanting the two electrodes called for an even greater degree of precision and accuracy than the choosing of the location of the lesions in the first operation, and it had to be done in as sterile environment as possible to minimize the possibility of rejection. The electrodes were to penetrate the brain by about six inches, at mid head to just below the nose and below the eye.

We were now about nine-and-a-half hours into the operation itself, sixteen hours since I had woken up, and over twenty hours since I had been taken off my meds. This procedure called for stamina and endurance that was stretching my resources to the limit.

It was exhausting for the surgeons too. Of the team of three, two were in the operating room at all times, along with the neurophysiologist and the neuropsychologist.

At the critical moment in the surgery, I had to urinate. I held off as long as I could, so much so that I was shaking. Lozano and Tasker were implanting the electrodes. Under no circumstances could my head move or the whole procedure would be compromised. "Let him pee his pants," said Lozano.

There had been a shift change and the OR was short-staffed. Jan Duff, Dr. Lang's trial co-ordinator, and Dr. Nestor Galvez, his clinical fellow, were pressed into service as nurses, but they didn't know where to find a bed pan. They almost made it, but not quite. As the warm urine flooded over me, I felt a combination of anger and humiliation. The surgeons' concern was to keep the open area of my brain sterile and uncontaminated—they were the focus of my anger at the humiliation of wetting my bed for the first time in over forty years. In a perverse way, it was positive, because it took my mind off the operation and the change in focus somehow gave me new energy.

I felt no effect from implanting the electrodes, probably due to a combination of physical exhaustion, the bed-wetting, and brain fatigue from all the prodding and poking. After the electrodes were inserted, Dr. Munz closed me up, a simple matter, and the operation was over. It had been twelve hours since they had begun fitting the stereotaxic frame on me.

The aftermath of the second operation was totally unlike the first. When I was wheeled into the recovery room, Esther, Howard, and Emily were there together with Pete Paterson and Stephen Booth. I held up my hand in a defiant Churchillian "V", but I did not feel victorious. I burst into tears. I was completely exhausted and, unlike the first operation, I had no sense of whether or not the operation had been a success.

I was in the recovery room for over an hour. I tried to sit up, but I could not. I was so tired that my body would not respond. With the intense weariness came a feeling of depression, a feeling that carried over to the next day. My overriding feeling was exhaustion instead of exhilaration. I had not been prepared for anything but good news or victorious feelings.

For most of the day after surgery, I felt exhausted and depressed. Since the operation, part of my face seemed to be paralyzed and I had a most unattractive drool. Several different groups of doctors had appeared to hook up the probes in my brain to a stimulator, all with indifferent results.

At the end of the day, Dr. Tasker, wearing his ever-present turtleneck sweater, appeared at my bedside with a stimulator and asked how the day had gone. "Not well" was the only response I could manage. I had come to appreciate the balding slightly portly man whose avocation is ornithology.

He hooked up the stimulator. I groaned to myself, "not more of this." He tried only a few settings. Then, a buddha-like look of inner peace came over his face as he said, "You'll be alright. It works!"

It was the first reassurance I'd had and the first moment of optimism after the operation. Those few words of encouragement carried me for a week.

The practical implications of the post-operative trauma were generalized facial swelling, transitory facial paralysis that caused my drool, and some problems with gait. As a result, my face felt puffy, I couldn't control my swallowing very well, hence the drool, and I felt funny walking. The psychological effect of this trauma on me and my family was substantial. I had accepted the high level of risk in the operation, but had not been prepared for these frustrating, ambiguous after-effects. I don't know if they had been anticipated by the doctors.

Because there was so much post-operative swelling, Dr. Peter Ashby, the physician who was doing the electrophysiological measurements, was concerned that the data he was getting was inaccurate and of limited utility. He decided that it would be necessary to bury the electrodes below the surface of my skull for six weeks. All the brain cell recording and the poking and prodding of the brain had taken a toll; I needed a rest to recuperate. On December 23, the leads to the electrodes were buried under my scalp to ensure that they would not be contaminated while my brain got back to normal.

In the days following the operation, I realized that there was considerable reduction in the muscular rigidity that came from my Parkinson's. I was able to cut back my daily dosage of Sinemet CR and Pergolide very substantially. This was an unexpected bonus of the operation. When the two electrodes were inserted in my left globus pallidus and sub-thalamic nucleus, my brain cells were moved, but not destroyed. This movement, though tiny, was enough to alter the brain's electrical circuitry in much the same way as the pallidotomy did in the first operation. No one knew how long these benefits would last, but the doctors thought they would be in addition to the benefits that would be obtained through chronic stimulation.

On December 24 I went home for Christmas, determined to enjoy the season with Esther, Howard, and Emily and our friends. That evening, while watching TV, I had a brain seizure, akin to a grand mal epileptic seizure. It lasted less than a minute, but I was left unconscious for hours. Nell West, Esther's cousin who is a nurse with the V.O.N., and who was staying with us, did all the right things, while my daughter Emily called 911. In no time, police car, fire department rescue truck, and ambulance were at our door and I was rushed to the Western.

Some friends had been dropping off a gift at our house on their way to the midnight service at Christ Church Deer Park when all the emergency vehicles were in front of our house. Word of my seizure traveled quickly during the service. Dozens of concerned friends called to see what the problem was.

Esther, Howie, Emily, and Nell had followed me down to the hospital in Nell's car. Fortunately, when I was being admitted, a doctor from the neurology department who happened to be familiar with my case was on duty. He made sure that the emergency room staff were aware that I was having post-operative problems (no doubt compounded by being too active) rather than thinking I was suffering from epilepsy.

Beyond the effect of the seizure on me, the major concern was whether anything had happened to the electrodes. The doctors were able to establish that nothing had gone wrong. I was still unconscious, but the doctors decided that my condition was stable. Unknown to me, in the emergency room Emily held my hand constantly. Everyone was exhausted and Esther eventually persuaded the rest of the family that there was nothing more they could do for me and they all left for home. Once there, they opened their Christmas stockings before they went to bed; they weren't expecting me home for a few days.

I don't know what time I woke up. No, that is incorrect. The right words are regained consciousness. I think it was late morning, and Howie was by my side. "Hi, what am I doing here? I left this bloody place. Why am I back here?" I had no idea of what had happened to me, no memory of my seizure. In fact I had no memory of what I was doing at the time. I have permanent amnesia of the moment leading up to the seizure.

I wanted to get up from my hospital bed, but Howie told me I must not. I did nonetheless, and fell a couple of times.

"Under no circumstances will you tell the nurses or doctors that I've fallen," I said to Howard. "If they found out, I'd never get out of this godforsaken place"

Poor Howie was torn. Esther had said to him, "Your father is to stay in the hospital as long as is necessary."

A resident doctor told me that I had had a "neurological incident," and would have to be very careful and quiet for some time. I was released about noon on Christmas Day with a prescription for a drug that was expected to prevent future seizures. Howie drove me home.

As I walked through the front door, the first thing I said was "what about the scrambled eggs and smoked salmon we always have for Christmas breakfast?" Esther, Nell, and Emily greeted me with relief. Then I sprung into action, completely ignoring the advice the doctors at the Western had given me about taking it easy.

Esther and Shannon Graham had predicted that something like this might happen, so they each had a turkey; only the vegetables had to be divvied up for our separate Christmas dinners. We had a post-Christmas dinner with them on the 28th and went to a large party with the Pearces, Vanstones, and Patersons on the 29th.

In the following couple of weeks, I had a serious depression. How long would the traumatic side effects last, or would they be permanent? Why was there no immediate benefit as there was after the first operation? Had the surgeons screwed up? There had been no pre-surgical counseling on any of my post-surgical problems. The discussions I had had with the doctors had been focused on the "big" things that could have gone wrong: rupturing a blood vessel, cognitive impairment, vision problems, and speech deterioration.

However, within a month, the signs of post-surgical trauma were gone, the benefits of the direct contact with the buried electronic probes continued, and I was a happy camper again.

On February 5, I went back to the Western for a week of electrophysiological tests to determine the appropriate settings for the pacemaker that was to be connected to the electrodes that were implanted in December. For the entire period, I was taken off my medication to enable the testers to determine the effect of stimulation in isolation. This reduced my mobility, but not nearly as much as I expected. In fact, to my surprise, I found I was reasonably mobile, much more so than I had been before the operation when my meds were off.

First, the wires that had been buried on December 23rd had to be bared. The operation was a simple one, but inevitably accompanied by a good deal of anxiety.

Once the wires were bared, initial tests made by Dr. Ashby determined that the reduced swelling in my brain made a significant difference to the responsiveness of the sub-thalamic nucleus and the globus pallidus. This good news resulted in my feeling a bit euphoric at the end of the first day.

There were two electrodes to be tested for my response to stimulation. In the initial testing by Dr. Ashby in December immediately after the operation, I was much more responsive to the subthalamic nucleus electrode. This time around, I was too responsive for the stimulator: at very low levels of stimulation, a 0.1 volt difference in amplitude or 10 hertz in frequency was enough to induce a quite painful contraction on the right side of my body. Hence, the neurologist and neurosurgeons decided not to connect the STN electrode, neither would they remove it; doing that would risk moving the brain cells in the GPI.

The rest of the week in hospital was lonely, tiring, and often frustrating. Lonely because Esther, with her MS, could not easily come down to the hospital more than once or twice. Howie and Emily came down almost every day and I loved seeing them and also the friends who visited. But they could not replace Esther whom I missed terribly.

Tiring because with each of the eighteen settings of the GPI electrode, the voltage would start at a low level, two volts, increasing by half a volt with each iteration, holding frequency and pulse width constant. Then voltage was held constant, and either frequency or pulse width varied. That meant a minimum of one hundred separate settings. With each setting, Nestor Galvez, the Clinical Fellow who was the testing neurologist, and the nurse who was doing the scoring, would put me through my paces on the Unified

Parkinson's Disease Rating Scale, testing for rigidity, flexibility, speech, mobility, and gait and balance among other things, to measure the effects of stimulation.

Frustrating because for 90 percent of the week, up to Friday afternoon, the stimulator was not producing any noticeable effect. I felt no improvement when it was turned on.

I was bound and determined that the stimulation was going to succeed. On Friday afternoon, when the last settings were tried, they worked, or at least I thought they did. Nestor disagreed. He said, "Bill, there is not enough difference to warrant permanent stimulation. I am going to recommend to Dr. Lang and Dr. Lozano that we not proceed with implanting the receiver—there will be no permanent stimulation."

I was crushed. Instant depression. All that I had put up with and endured up to that point seemed to be for nothing.

It was a tough call that Nestor made because there were a lot of people at the hospital who were hoping that stimulation would be successful, in particular the team of Lang, Lozano, Tasker, and Jan Duff. But Dr. Galvez called it as he saw it.

Dr. Lozano came to my bedside at about 6:30 Friday evening with his neurosurgical fellow to give me the bad news.

"But Andres, it works!" I argued.

"That's not what Dr. Galvez says."

"I felt the difference. In the last setting we tried."

"Prove it," said Lozano, sceptically. "What setting were you on?"

"Two negative and three positive at 180 hertz and a pulse width of one hundred micro seconds."

Lozano hooked me up, using a frequency of 450 hertz because Dr. Ashby's previous work suggested a higher frequency might produce better results.

Like Lazarus, I walked, first in my hospital room, then in the corridor. Surprised disbelief replaced the sad look on Andres' face.

"Let's see if you can make it to Dr. Lang's office."

I was excited. The bloody thing was working! I put on my dressing gown and slippers and walked. Past the nursing station, then to the central corridor in the hospital. I was across the long passageway between two of the hospital buildings. Then into an elevator, up six floors to Dr. Lang's office. With just the stimulator on.

"Pretty convincing," said Lozano, enthusiastically.

Determination counts. If I had just meekly accepted the first conclusion, the doctors would have abandoned the attempt at electronic deep brain stimulation and I would not have experienced the full benefit of the operation.

As it was, during the post-operative testing, I was off my medications totally for four days—longer than I could have previously imagined possible. The remarkable thing was that I was on the verge of being on without any medication at all. This was a consequence of the brain cells being moved when the probes were being inserted and is a lasting benefit of the operation.

The end of testing was in sight, but it would not be reached until the pacemaker was successfully implanted and operational. The testing and waiting ... and testing ... and waiting ... were tedious and frustrating.

There are pluses and minuses to being a medical first. On the one hand there is the excitement of being a pioneer; on the other is the time it takes to make sure that everything is being done properly. On that the medical team would not compromise, nor should they. Too much was at stake.

Because deep brain stimulation was a new technique there was no standard-issue electronic pacemaker for me to use. Pacemaker technology was originally developed to deal with hearts that were arrhythmic; consequently the fully implantable models have the limitations of being designed for cardiac purposes—for instance the maximum frequency is 180 hertz. I would need at least 220 hertz with a pulse width of 200 milliseconds. Medtronic, Inc., a leading supplier, has adapted the cardiac technology to deal with neurological problems such as intractable pain and Parkinson's-related problems. Medtronic's ingenious interim solution was to develop an external transmitter that has an antenna placed directly over a receiver implanted under the collarbone. The receiver then transmits the stimulation via wires tunneled down the side of the neck from the electrodes at the top of the head.

The system was hooked up on March 3, 1995. Since that day, my life has been transformed for a second time.

CHAPTER ELEVEN

An End and Beginning

The effect of the second operation, combined with the first, was truly dramatic and miraculous for me. People in our neighbourhood whom I didn't know but who had observed me, stopped me on the street and said "What has happened to you? There is such a tremendous change in you!" I was and am, to borrow a phrase from C.S. Lewis, "surprised by joy": by the joy of freedom. Freedom to do what I want to do, within reasonable limits.

The operations were not a cure for my Parkinson's. That is not possible yet. But the worst of my symptoms are under control. My Parkinsonian mask is gone, my arms swing naturally when I walk, and my walking is vastly improved. On the minus side, my speech is a bit worse, my handwriting is hopeless, and I tire more easily. When I am overtired, my speech becomes unintelligible, mobility deteriorates, and co-ordination can be a real problem. That's the challenge: to know when to stop, and then to stop.

I still take four Sinemet CRs per day, and I try to take them on time. Before my first operation I was taking fourteen of those blessed pills each day, one every two and half hours, and even then I could never tell when I would become completely immobilized.

I no longer take a cane with me when I leave the house, to Esther's relief. I used to walk with my cane outstretched behind me, but after I caught a young woman and later a small child between the legs, Esther dared not take her eyes off me while we walked. The cane was more like a gelding instrument. I am now a free man ... well, not really free because I now have to have my little portable stimulator hooked up all my waking hours. It is no larger than a Walkman, but it consumes one 9-volt Duracell battery every day.

I am able to live a normal life. I look like a normal person. I am no longer the frightening-looking person whose violent shaking alarmed and repelled people. I no longer feel or am perceived to be alienated from society. When I get up in the morning I take our very lively Airedale terrier on a five-kilometre walk. I have been re-certified to drive a car. I go to meetings, go out to lunch. We travel.

For the first summer after the operation, at Blue Sea Lake I prepared for water sports by buying a waterproof bag to safeguard the pacemaker when I was sailing or canoeing. It turned out that the main danger was not getting it wet, but having it bang around in the sailboat when coming about or gybing. I tried, somewhat apprehensively, going out without the pacemaker. To my surprise and delight, I found that, as long as my pills have been taken on time, doing without a pacemaker is not a problem. My movements and agility are not quite as good as with the pacemaker, but are more than adequate. On the matter of golf, while I have only played half a dozen games in my life, I can now drive a ball seventy-five to one hundred yards; the difference is that the ball often lands in the middle of the fairway instead of everywhere but.

Looking back over the operations, I realize that despite the very legitimate apprehension about the dangers of a bilateral pallidotomy, it seems that the mini-pallidotomy and sub-thalamotomy that had to be performed in the second operation to insert the electrodes had the most beneficial effect on my condition, and that the electronic stimulator is, most of the time, the icing on the cake. I have gone for most of a morning without medication and just the stimulator. With the stimulator alone, I am not as well off as with both, but I can function well enough to take public transit to the hospital for testing.

The physical and practical improvements are dramatic. Apart from the sheer pleasure of living close to a normal life, there is the relief of being able to help Esther. Because of her condition, I had to be mobile if we were to be able to live our lives together. This is the great practical benefit. I am able to look after the household. Not only that, we can travel together. I can get her on a train or plane.

I believe in miracles. At Easter, 1995, I wrote a poem, Miracles, to try to set down my feelings about my operations. It is a sort of postscript to Lazarus:

MIRACLES

A child healed because a prayer has been said
Or a sacrifice offered to a household god
Or because a different doctor is consulted
Is not a miracle.
A child could just as well die from these things.

An apparition can be the result of an altered state of mind
Brought about by pain or hunger or fatigue or mortification.
Or by the magic mushroom or peyote-mescaline.
Not a miracle, just hallucination
Self-induced, deliberate escape.

An auto-stigmatizing statue or one that cries
The Lady's tears of pain
Is often a calculated attempt
To deceive the faithful
or one's self.

Honest piety, judiciously applied to human endeavour
Can produce things that pass human understanding;
But these are not miracles.
For they require a special talent

Like the shaman in The Cunning Man.

Miracles involve perceptions of reality
Different from the everyday interpretation
Of what makes life tick on.
A miracle-worker is not
An ordinary human.

They are well-schooled in their art-form
They aren't ordinary whiz kids.
They dazzle with their insights
Us ordinary folk
Who aren't in their league.

Super-tuned and extra-focused ears and eyes
Interpreting reality differently
Neurons and receptors arrhythmically conversing.
Discovering why there is disorder and chaos
Is the miracle.

For they have been there always.
Waiting to be discovered by human senses
They elude the common mind
The idler's tongue
They are not invented.

They are the apogee of Creation.
When understood in their fullness
Miracles explain the mysteries
Of the world in human terms
To human beings.

The definition of miracles I arrive at in my poem frees me from the doctrinaire position that if it did not happen in the Bible, it is not part of God's revelation. It permits—no, insists—that the insights of Einstein and Freud be part of God's world. The special skills of the modern scientist combine finely honed perceptions with lateral thinking. These skills are fired in the crucible of technology, for these finer perceptions would not be possible without the benefits of science, and it is these finer perceptions that allow scientists to perform miracles. I believe in miracles because I have had two miracles worked on me.

There is a real sense in which the effects of these operations remain a mystery. Medical science knows how lesions affect the brain and how chronic stimulation affects movement, but as the philosopher John Searle observed,

> As far as we know the relevant processes take place at themicro levels of synapses, neurons and cell assemblies. All our conscious life is caused by these lower level processes, but we have only the foggiest idea of how it all works.[8]

We know how the motor system works, but we do not know how the neurobiological processes in the brain cause consciousness. The answer to the question of consciousness is tied up with the old philosophical problem of dualism: the placing of consciousness and other mental phenomena outside the ordinary world and thus outside the scope of natural science.

Opponents of this view argue that dualism must be abandoned and we should start with the assumption that consciousness is an ordinary biological phenomena like digestion or growth.

The two operations I had were tremendously successful and I get great satisfaction from writing and speaking about them. But I know that these risky medical procedures are only suitable for a small proportion of those who suffer from Parkinson's, or other chronic neurological conditions. The neurosurgical/medical team chose me to be their guinea pig, in part because I was comparatively young, and I was, except for Parkinson's (and that is quite a big "except for") in quite good psychological and physical health, and had no other chronic medical conditions that could adversely affect the outcome.

Not long after my second operation, I saw the results of another bilateral pallidotomy that had been done in two separate procedures a year apart. The patient, a man in his sixties, was a diabetic. After the second procedure, he was left with severe gait, cognitive, and balance problems. The tragic experience of this patient is compounded by the agony his family must endure.

Another factor that restricts pallidotomies being used widely for the treatment of Parkinson's is that these operations require such a high level of medical and technical skill that it may be unrealistic to propose that all those thousands of patients in Canada alone who might benefit from the operations should have them. However, in the four and a half years since the second operation my medication costs have been reduced by over fifty thousand dollars, so there could be an economic argument for the operation.

For a patient, making the decision to undergo brain surgery of this sort is difficult and frightening, for the outcomes of these operations can vary dramatically. In the years since my operations quite a large number of people have undergone the same procedure with varying results. A number of them have told their stories on a website. (<http://www.geocities.com/SoHo/Village/6263/pienet/hithgang/index.html>.) Some are ecstatically happy, others disappointed or frustrated. It would be unwise to draw firm conclusions from this anecdotal evidence, but it is clear that the important factors for success are the physical and emotional condition of the patient and the quality and experience of the surgeons. Reading these stories makes me appreciate all the more how fortunate I was.

On November 27, 2000 Esther and I attended Dr. Ron Tasker's retirement dinner. As the only patient invited, I felt very honoured. There were neurosurgeons from Japan, Brazil, Europe and America who had come considerable distances to pay tribute to Ron, their doyen. I said:

> Let there be no doubt! I owe my life to Ron Tasker. He performed two procedures on me: a pallidotomy in December, 1993 and a Deep Brain

> Stimulation, the first in North America just a year later. As you might imagine, the day after the second operation I wasn't feeling exactly 100% after all the poking and prodding in my brain—I imagine you neurosurgeons have a more elegant term for it than that. At about six o'clock in the evening a Bhudda-like figure appeared at my bedside. It was Ron. He was wearing a grey turtle neck sweater, with his glasses suspended from his neck by the same red cord they are this evening. He took a neurostimulator out of his pocket and tried a few settings. "It works. You'll be alright!" Those words of assurance carried me through weeks of testing and fine tuning. Six years have passed. It still works and I'm still alright. Thank-you Ron, for restoring me to a normal life.

The operations that were performed on me are only one approach to the treating of Parkinson's. In effect, the pallidotomies with deep brain stimulation are an acknowledgement that a part of the nervous system is irrevocably broken. Another treatment approach is along the line of dopamine replacement. My only experiences of this are the medications Pergolide and Sinemet CR. Now, a whole new generation of dopamine agonists is being developed, and there is great pressure to make them available to patients before they have been thoroughly tested. One of these drugs has had to be removed from the market because of fatal adverse reactions in some patients.

Fetal transplants have long been the dream of neurologists and neurosurgeons. Technically, this procedure is a form of organ transplant, but in terms of treatment for Parkinson's it is an extension of dopamine replacement therapy. At present, it raises difficult practical and ethical questions. In order to treat each side of a patient's brain, six or eight voluntarily aborted six-to eight week old fetuses are needed. If this treatment were to become widely used, the number of fetuses required would give the most ardent abortion free-choicer pause. Fetal transplants were first attempted in the 1970s and techniques have developed quickly since then, however slowly it seems to desperate Parkinsonians. Results of a recent double blind study were very positive and parallel the results of other types of surgery. But it must be admitted that all these procedures are based on what the noted physician Lewis Thomas calls "halfway technologies." He does not use the term derisively, but to point out that they do not represent a cure, only better symptom management.

In the years since my operations, much of my time has been spent working with the administration and work of the Parkinson's Foundation, as well as the peer support programme. Among the projects I've been involved in are the growth of the SuperWalk, the initiation and development of the peer support programmes, as well as sitting on the board and on various committees. I have also attended international

Parkinson's conferences. In effect I have become a professional Parkinsonian.

My neurosurgical experience has been the great adventure of my life. Imagine the thrill of having your brain operated on twice, each time fully awake. And the predicted results happened: I have been born again. Not in the sense of religion, but in being free to move and act. My life is ahead of me.

People have said that I am an inspiration and a hero to them. I find such statements profoundly embarrassing, because I have done nothing that is heroic or inspirational. I had no choice. Without the two operations, I would be spending the rest of my life bedridden in an institution.

I know that in our family I am the lucky one. Esther's condition has progressed considerably (in medical terminology) in the seven years since her diagnosis. Her gait and balance have deteriorated as a result of two factors not directly related to multiple sclerosis. In the summer of 1995 she broke her right hip, and there has been a development of chronic pain in her left shoulder and neck that radiates to her feet and hands. This pain is so severe as to be debilitating and has rendered her a semi-invalid. A whole arsenal of drug therapy has been tried with only limited success. In the first place, the so-called pain-killers don't kill pain, they only take the edge off. And they have adverse side effects ranging from weight-gain to worsening coordination. There is the possibility that neuro-surgery similar to deep brain stimulation could alleviate the pain, although at present the success rate for this treatment is only about fifty percent.

Even with the 50/50 odds of the deep brain stimulation being successful, Esther had the operation on September 14, 2000. For her, it was a nine-hour procedure. It took so long because the part of the thalmus that regulates pain is extremely difficult to locate. There were two periods of testing in the hospital; her neurostimulator was implanted and installed on February 19, 2001. The surgical staples will be removed on February 28, with the stimulator being activated that day. We are anticipating success!

What is it about us, as a family, that causes us to go to the brink of incapacity and then choose surgical intervention, experimental and at the leading edge of technology and the limit of human knowledge?

We have tried all the available drug therapies and they have not proven satisfactory, either because they don't work or because they produce intolerable side effects. There is nothing left except experimental surgery. The alternative is incarceration in a long-term care facility, with the world cut off from us and we being cut off from the world.

We are exceedingly fortunate to have Dr. Andres M. Lozano as our neurosurgeon, the leading functional neurosurgeon in practice today. He is a miracle worker who thrives on challenges that push him to the limit of his capabilities. He makes neurosurgery the clear choice.

One morning in May 1999, our son Howie, who was now twenty-eight, phoned us from Vancouver where he was studying, to say that his ulcerative colitis was excruciatingly painful. We could hear the pain in the sound of his voice. He had been suffering from this condition for several years—it was the consequence of drinking bad water on a canoe trip. Ulcerative colitis is a chronic disease of the bowel characterized by sores or ulcers on the inner surface of the large intestine that are extremely painful. Digestion becomes difficult and there is a lack of control over bowel movements. These features combined with the medication he was taking having become toxic had caused Howie to become less gregarious and somewhat reclusive.

Howie told us that he had an appointment with his gastroenterologist the next afternoon. We urged him not to wait but to go to Emergency at once. He did, and that afternoon he was in St. Paul's Hospital in Vancouver with emergency surgery, an ileostomy, scheduled for the next evening. In the end four feet—about one and a quarter metres of Howie's large intestine—would be removed.

I got the first available flight to Vancouver to be with Howie. As I walked into his hospital at noon the day after his operation he was asleep. I said, "Howie, it's Dad. I'm here." He woke up, surprised to see me.

Tears welled up in my eyes as we hugged each other. I felt very vulnerable.

Over the next week as we talked, I was thrilled by Howie's positive attitude. One statement of his hit home. "I'm regaining control of my life!"

The true dread of everyone who has a chronic disease is the lack of control they have over their life. Where once our lives had been run by our diseases we had had—first I and then Howie—leading-edge technology surgery. We have been doubly blessed with a second chance at life. What we make of it will determine if we are worthy.

With chronic disease you have to be angry enough with the disease that you say, "I will not permit this condition to run my life any more." But you must not only have been diagnosed with a chronic illness, you must experience it yourself for a period of time—for everyone's experience is different. As Nietzsche wrote,

> He who seeth the abyss, but with the eagle's eye—he who with the eagle's talons graspeth the abyss: he hath courage.

You must go to the edge of the abyss, look in and decide that this is not the future you want. In T.S. Eliot's play Murder in the Cathedral, the chorus says,

> We are afraid in a fear which we cannot know, which we cannot face which none understands, And our hearts are torn from us, our brains

> unskinned like the layers of an onion, ourselves are lost in a final fear which none understands.

And that surely is the point. No one who has seen the bottom of the abyss wants to be there. Hope must never be abandoned.

APPENDIX A

My Case Report

THE QUALITY OF LIFE IS WHAT COUNTS

BY WILLIAM A. HARSHAW[9] MY STORY

I am one of the fortunate ones. I was diagnosed with Parkinson's disease on a miserable February day twenty years ago. I have lived to tell my story. Seven years ago I couldn't walk.

Imagine, if you can, being unable to control your body, being utterly immobilized. I found an account by Oliver Sacks, about another situation, that described my feelings well:

> The leg was in exile ... or it was not where it should be. Normally we are so at home in our bodies and we so own them that things like this are unimaginable.[10]

It didn't strike me at the time, but my initial experience with Parkinson's disease was much like Albert Camus' great postwar novel La Chute and Dante Alighieri's Inferno, an exploration of Hell. Now, we have recently been told by the Bishop of Rome that Hell is not spatially located in our Universe, but is a state of mind in which we are separated from God. If that is true, and it must be for it was an *ex cathedra pronunciamento,* it must be like advanced

Parkinson's disease. If you have advanced Parkinson's disease, it is more than imaginable: it is reality.

I spent the first four years of my life with PD in denial, one of the most foolish things one can do. I "came out" in the spring of1985 at a lunch party that I was holding for a group that had financially supported a candidate in the provincial election that year. One of the guests came up to me and said: "That must be one Hell of a hangover you're nursing, Bill!" I was shocked at my response:"That's no hangover, Douglas, I have Parkinson's disease." I hadn't planned to come out, but it was long overdue. I later wondered why I had waited so long!

If I had not had two highly successful experimental neurosurgical procedures, one in each of 1993 and 1994, I would be incarcerated in a long-term care facility and would likely have died by now.

I have come to realize that, for me, Parkinson's disease is a gift and is the great liberating influence in my life. I do not make this statement lightly. The remainder of this article will, in a very imprecise way, quantify that statement and explain the way the numbers are derived.

Before my operations, it slowly dawned on me that as I became more physically constrained by Parkinson's disease, my mind was not at all constrained. During those hours when I couldn't move, I read voraciously and listened to classical music and jazz. It was a time of spiritual and intellectual liberation. I wrote the following lines of poetry at that time:

> Mornings were a dull routine.
> Immobile.
> Many hours would pass until my brain's command
> My anxious limbs its tortured message reached.
> And permitted steps, first halting
> Like a child would take.
> Then runstumble.
> Strangers asked:
> "What troubles him?
> His legs like branches on a misshaped tree
> Do move in deformed harmony."

There is little doubt that Parkinson's disease has the potential to be physically, emotionally, and financially crippling for patients and their families. This sad truth is paradoxical because more has been discovered by research scientists and the medical profession in the way of palliative—not curative—therapies than is the situation for any other neuro degenerative disease. Indeed, media reports of neurosurgery performed on Parkinson's patients in the last decade tend to have an almost Lourdes-like quality about them. It is instructive to quote the from the American novelist Willa Cather's Death Comes for the Archbishop:

> ...Miracles ... seem to me to rest not so much upon faces or voices or healing power coming suddenly near to us from afar off, but upon our perceptions being made finer, so that for a

> moment our eyes can see and our ears can hear what is there about us always.[11]

The recent advances in neurosurgical instrumentation and diagnostic imaging are really nothing more than extensions of the surgeon's five senses: touch, sight, hearing, taste, and smell, making their perceptions finer. This heightening of perceptions comes at a high cost, with anything that is high technology and medical being very expensive.

A new neurosurgical procedure—the implantation of electrodes in my basal ganglia, a brain structure located in the middle of the brain about level with the bottom of my nose—followed by passing electric current through the electrode produced a dramatic easing of my Parkinson's symptoms. The improvement was so great that I have called the time after the procedure "my second chance at life." The controlled use of electric current has been an effective therapeutic intervention for many medical conditions, ranging from irregular heart beat and chronic pain to severe depression and Parkinson's disease and incontinence ... the list could go on.

My life is my own again. To the extent that any of us are, I am in control again. My balance and walking are greatly improved and slowness and poverty of movement are a thing of the past. When I get up in the morning, I turn on my neurostimulator, take my medication and go for a brisk five kilometre walk with my five-year-old Airedale Terrier, "Madam." That was not possible before.

The remainder of this article will focus on the economic evaluation of DBS as a palliative therapy for Parkinson's disease. Over the past five years, I had often wondered about trying to marry the obvious improvements in my quality of life and the easing of my Parkinsonian symptoms with the economics of the procedure. I found myself in a brave new world where, to purists, everything is reduced to statistics and the human element does not enter the decision-making process.

THE CASE REPORT: ECONOMIC EVALUATION

In working on this project, I was very conscious of an aphorism by my great-great uncle Sir William Osler, the eminent physician, medicine is a vocation in which the heart is exercised equally with the head. I could not permit a medicrat's solution to be my conclusion.

As I looked into the evolving discipline, subspecialties like biostatistics, sample design, clinical epidemiology, and survey questionnaire design were ones that came up frequently. And then there were the different types of economic analysis: cost effectiveness, cost utility, and cost benefit. How could anyone not in the business make sense of it? If this was not a priesthood of believers; it was not dissimilar to a secret society with passwords and mantras.

Economics, I remembered from my introductory course in the subject, was called the "dismal science" by the nineteenth century Scottish historian Thomas Carlyle. While, as a discipline, it has evolved considerably since Victorian England, economics is still concerned with the allocation of scarce resources between competing ends. Health Care Economics helps clarify the trade-offs involved in policy formulation. David Naylor, the Dean of Medicine at the University of Toronto, in a 1996 article[12] recommends that, when using the results of economic analysis we should:

> temper ... interpretations with common sense, leavened by compassion and a sense of justice.

The questions I am going to try to answer are:

1. How are the changes in a patient's quality of life measured?
2. How is the change in the patient's medical condition measured?
3. How are the answers to the first two questions used to determine the cost per unit of change?

The first thing to understand is that this is can be made into a highly complex business. For example, you don't just ask an individual "How much did your quality of life improve as a result of the operation?" and make your assessment based on the answer. One of the reasons is that people have a general desire to describe their experience in as positive a light as possible. So the questions have to be asked in such a way as to elicit unbiased responses and to ensure that the participants are being consistent in their answers..

Likewise with the sample of participants in the survey. Asking just one patient and basing the assessment on his answers could be misleading because the one patient might be unrepresentative in age, background socio-economic status or medical condition. The sample must be designed so that it is just the right size and composition. For instance in a condition affecting age groups in a specific way, it would make sense to have the sample reflect the demographics of the disease.

To use another example, if gross changes are being examined, a smaller sample size is needed than if subtle changes are being looked for, the reason being that nuances are often difficult to detect.

In a clinical trial there are typically two subsets of the participants: the control group, which does not receive the new therapy, but instead gets either a placebo or another drug; and the test group, which gets the therapy being tested.. If two therapies are being tested for relative effectiveness, the double blind[13] will be applied to three possibilities: therapy A, therapy B and a control, therapy C.

When the questions have been asked of the sample, the data must be analyzed very carefully to insure that the data does not yield in correct inferences. This process is complex and time consuming. The statistical analysis is exhaustive to the point of being nit-picky. Why, you might very well ask, do they push the numbers so far? The only answer is because human lives depend upon the outcome.

It makes no sense to perform an economic evaluation on an intervention that has been shown to be clinically ineffective. If a thing isn't worth doing, it isn't worth doing well. That is not to say that carefully designed classic clinical evaluations should not be carried out for most interventions. Far from it. They are the only way to definitively establish effectiveness.

1. How are changes in a patient's quality of life measured?

They are measured in terms of QALY, an acronym that stands for Quality- Adjusted Life Year. The idea of QALY is to come up with an estimate of how long a patient's life has been extended and how much his quality of life has altered. For example, a patient with cancer whose life span has been shortened by five years and whose quality of life would have gone down from 0.9 to 0.25 without treatment could say that cancer had cost him 3.25 QALYs. Any strategy to improve his quality of life to, say 0.6, for an improvement of 1.5 QALYs and cost $100,000 would cost $65,000 per QALY When a health care intervention is made in a person's life, a series of carefully prepared questions will be put to the patient. Typically, the response to each question is scored from zero to one, with zero representing death and one representing perfect health. It is possible to have a negative score for life being worse than death. Not all questions are of equal importance, so the answers are weighted to reflect their significance.

Table 1: QALYs

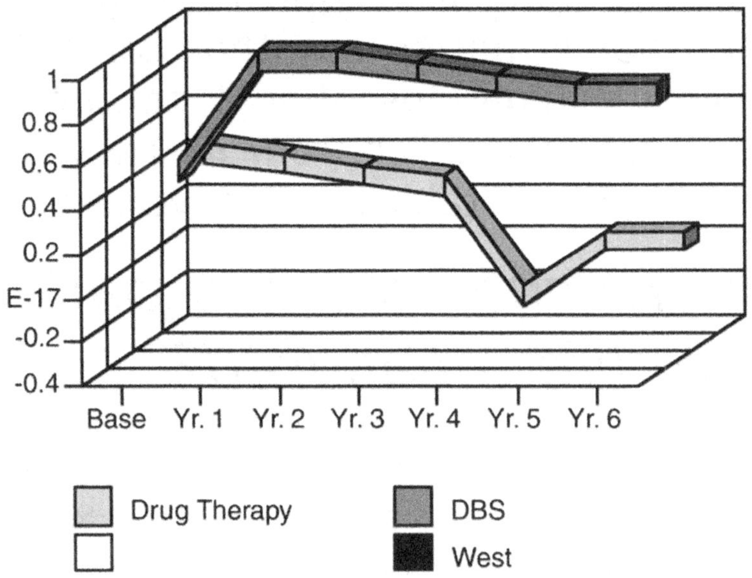

	Drugs	DBS
Base	0.40	0.40
Year 1	0.35	0.90
Year 2	0 .30	0.90
Year 3	0.25	0.85
Year 4	-0.25	0.80
Year 5	0	0.75
Year 6	0	0.75
Total	1.05	5.35

In isolation, the results obtained are meaningless. A comparison must be chosen that is a reasonable alternative to the intervention being evaluated.

The intervention being evaluated is Deep Brain Stimulation ("D.B.S."), a new procedure, and the comparison is a drug therapy case with no intervention neurosurgically.

DBS involves the implantation of microelectrodes in either the thalmus, globus pallidus or the subthalamic nucleus and then applying chronic electrical stimulation to the relevant brain structure. It differs from the conventional thalamotomy or pallidotomy in that no brain tissue is destroyed.

Typically, neurosurgery is offered as a therapeutic option to patients whose drug response is slowing down and who are experiencing serious adverse effects from their anti-Parkinson medication to the extent that these effects are disabling. Many Persons with Advanced Parkinson's Disease ("PAPD") are not offered neurosurgery on account of other medical conditions, unrelated to PD, which render them unsuitable surgical candidates. Also they may be subject to dementia and/or cognitive problems as a result of PD . They remain on drug therapy. A consequence of this lack of alternatives is a continuation of, and possible worsening, of the adverse effects of medication. These can lead to more accidents in the home or out and about in the community. Often, a PAPD will become reclusive, not wanting to leave his home and not moving much in his home. PAPDs are admitted to hospital more frequently than the general population and they tend to stay longer.

For the comparison purposes of this article it is assumed that I remained on my prescribed regime before my operations for the five and half year study period until the beginning of year five when I die.[14] This is not an unrealistic scenario, nor is the assumption that I would enter a long-term care facility within six months of the study's commencement.

There are quality of life rating scales that are disease-specific and generic ones that have as their objective determining the extent to which patients being rated have had non-trivial changes in their quality of life. Both types have positive and negative attributes, and both types are useful, although in different situations.

2. How are the changes in the patient's medical condition measured?

There are a number of rating scales, of which the Unified Parkinson's Disease Rating Scale ("UPDRS") is the most widely used, that comprehensively rate the patient. It is often difficult to separate a patient's change in medical condition from changes in his quality of life. Rating patients is an art as much as a skill. The rater must be constantly alert to ensure that the evaluation of the patient is as bias-free as possible.

Under the no intervention scenario, my quality of life deteriorated to the extent that I believed that life was a fate worse than death. I entered a long-term care facility half-way through year one and died at the beginning of year five.

With DBS, however, I had a gain of 4.95 QALYs. The next step in the analysis is to calculate the annual cost of the two cases.

Table 2: Annual Cost (rounded to '000s)

	Drugs	DBS
Base	$19.9	$45.6
year 1	$25.6	$5.9
Year 2	$34.3	$6.1
Year 3	$34.3	$6.0
Year 4	$34.3	$6.1
Year 5	0	$6.5
Year 6	0	$7.4

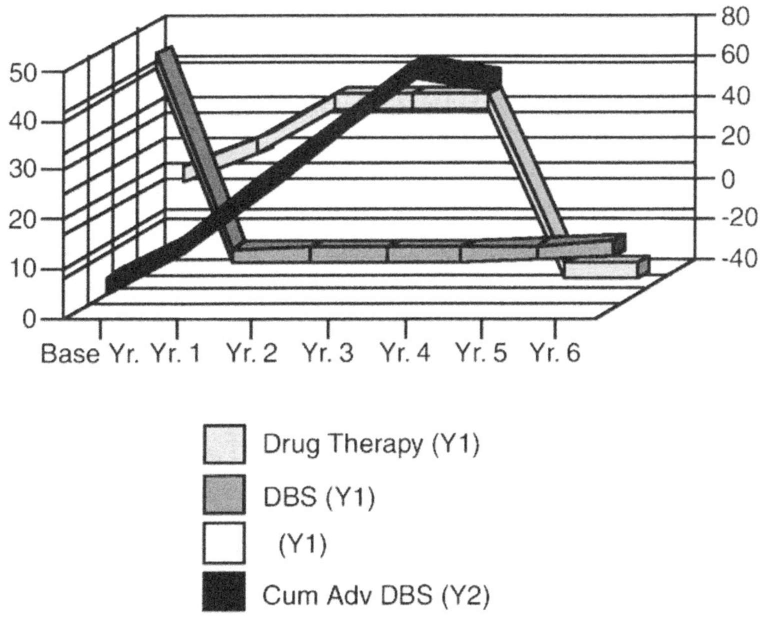

The mathematically inclined reader will note that in all charts the key is the area between the two lines. In Chart 1 the area between the lines is the number of QALYs gained by having the DBS procedure. In Chart 2, the area is the net financial benefit from having DBS rather than no neurosurgical intervention.

Looking at the two charts together, we see that there is a net gain of 4.30 QALYs from having the DBS procedure rather than have noneurosurgical intervention. Interestingly, the expenditure of money to obtain this result is C$65,000 less than "no intervention," for a negative C$16,000 per QALY. Put another way, using a surgical procedure that is at the limit of human knowledge and uses the highest technology available is less expensive than drug therapy. Not only that, the patient's quality of life is ahead by more than 4.25 QALYs. Putting it yet another way, the DBS alternative generates positive cash flow over the life of the patient.

There is one thing remaining to do. The time value of money must be taken into account. This is best illustrated by using an example: Would you rather have one million dollars today or $1,000 a week for life. If you are 50 years old when you are presented with this choice, $1 million = $1 million. If you live to age 75, not an unreasonable assumption, $1,000 per week using a 5% discount factor, you will only have received $725,000. It's a question of jam today instead of jam tomorrow. Assume you die on day one of your 76th year, the company will pocket a profit of $175,000.[15] The person would have to complete his 86th year to come out ahead on this scheme.

The interesting point that comes out when the data is present valued is that in real, i.e. discounted terms, the cost of each therapeutic alternative remained roughly constant over the study period.

ANECDOTES FROM MY CASE FILE

Since my operations, much of my time has been spent working with the administration and work of the Parkinson's Foundation, as well as the Peer Support Programme. Among the projects I've been involved in are the growth of the SuperWalk (a fundraising event), the initiation and development of the Peer Support Programmes, and sitting on the Board and on various committees. I have also attended international Parkinson's conferences. In effect, I have become a professional Parkinsonian.

My neurosurgical experience has been the great adventure of my life. Imagine the thrill of having your brain operated on twice—each time fully awake. And the predicted results happened: I have been born again. Not in the sense of religion, but in being free to move and act. My life is ahead of me.

And now we are three.... Our family has had extraordinary good fortune. First me, then Howie and just last month, Esther have regained control of our lives through the miracle of leading edge, high-technology surgery. These procedures, in the words of Thomas Cranmer, the principal author of *The Book of Common Prayer,* have enabled us to "...cast away the works of darkness and put upon us the armour of light...." Thomas Mann, the great twentieth-century German novelist, says in his essay "The making of the Magic Mountain":

> ...one must go through the deep experience of sickness and death to arrive at a higher sanity and health, in just the same way that one must have a knowledge of sin in order to find redemption...[16]

Our respective nadirs have been bottomless pits into which disease has seduced us. It is all too easy to stay in the pit, falsely recognizing that while it is miserable there it is worse outside. Nothing could be further from the truth. A defining characteristic of abysses is that no light shines into them. The way out is not marked in anyway or fashion. It is so difficult to surmount the obstacles—there is no course to teach you how. Time after time, you will be tempted to stay; not that the abyss is in any way paradise, but that it is so difficult to get out that there cannot be a reason to have to conquer the moats unless the outside is infinitely better than the abyss. You must go to the edge of the abyss, look in and decide that while you are still capable of doing so, this is not the future you want. In T.S. Eliot's play *Murder in the Cathedral,* the chorus says,

> We are afraid in a fear which we cannot know, which we cannot face, which none understands, And our hearts are torn from us, our brains unskinned like the layers of an onion, ourselves are lost in a final fear which none understands.[17]

And that surely is the point. No one who has seen the bottom of the abyss wants to be there. Hope must never be abandoned.

ACCESS TO THERAPY

Esther, Howie, and I are the fortunate ones. We have been able to conquer our chronic diseases with a combination of will power, determination, and providence. And we have an uncanny ability to get to the head of the line. Dr. Tony Lang, my movement disorders neurologist, said to me in the Fall of 1992 when I told him of Esther's diagnosis with MS "We have a duty to keep you mobile as long as possible." Who have we bumped to get to the head of the line? I don't know, but we are guilty of a great sin of commission if we have caused anyone to wait unnecessarily for therapy.

The Canadian health care system is predicated on two basic assumptions: universal timely access; and that the patient's economic resources are not to be an issue in determining access to therapy. A two-tier system is expressly prohibited as is extra billing.

Granted, the system is forty years old and has not had a fundamental redesign since its incarnation; it has been like a patch work quilt or the "Curate's Egg." (A young curate was having breakfast with his bishop. When the bishop asked how his boiled egg was, the reply is alleged to have been: "Parts of it, My Lord, are excellent.")

There is an old aphorism in the legal business: "Access to justice delayed is access denied." That may be equally applied to medicine. David Alter and his colleagues at the Institute for Clinical Evaluative Sciences in Toronto have published two articles[18] in which they demonstrate that socioeconomic status counts. Eighty percent of cardiologists, cardiac surgeons, and hospital CEOs had been personally involved in managing a patient who had received preferential access on the basis of factors other than medical need. The difference between the lowest quintile in income levels and the highest in utilization of specialists is 23 percent while the difference in waiting time was 45 percent lower. They also found a strong inverse relationship between income levels and one year death rates: for every $10,000 in income, the risk of one year death rate declines by 10 percent.

These findings are not indicative of the crude, gross discrimination that a casual reading the data presented in the preceding paragraph suggests. I do not believe that money changes hands—no filthy lucre. The bias is, in fact likely far more pernicious and subtle. It can probably be safely assumed that income levels are directly proportional to educational achievement. The better educated one is, the more able (s) he is to both understand the issues and implications of the medical condition. And further, the more likely (s) he is to ask intelligent questions about the condition and the probable consequences of different therapies. As well, some physicians are more adept as advocates for their patients than are others.[19]

A "high-end" doctor is more likely to be a better advocate and have patients in the higher socioeconomic groups of society. Is a lack of education, relatively poor socioeconomic status combined with a physician who is a poor advocate reason enough to consign such individuals to the dung heap of substandard medical care?

Absolutely not! That is why Medtronic Inc. is investing US$100 million in WebMD, an internet resource for patients. WebMD will provide the inquiring patient with the information needed to ask the physician basic questions about his or her condition. This, however, does not address the issue of the computer illiterate.

While the Alter's surveys were conducted related solely with reference to cardiological issues, there is no reason to believe that neurologists and neurosurgeons would act in a different manner. In fact cardiologists have less reason to act in this fashion because there is a provincial registry listing all cardiac patients in order of priority.

Access to proven effective therapies is an "as of right" entitlement. To delay or deny is to cause unnecessary pain and suffering. In our society, this pain and suffering is intolerable. The only remedy in the short term is publicity. In the long term, education is the only answer

CONCLUSIONS

This project was begun as a comprehensive study of DBS from an economic standpoint. When I became aware of the time and resources that would be necessary to undertake such a study, I scaled back the scope of the project.

Economics are not the only consideration, but they are important. It is tempting to consider the higher up-front cost of DBS and discard it. To do that would ignore the long-term cost savings and the immense quality of life improvement. The whole picture must be considered, not just a detail that happens to coincide with a reader's bias.

What are the conclusions of my case report? First, the findings, which are purely anecdotal, and subject to all the limitations of non-randomized groups with n=1, should be validated by a peer-reviewed economic evaluation of D.B.S. Pending the commissioning and receipt of that report, the following tentative conclusions may be reached:

1. D.B.S. is an effective therapeutic intervention for patients with advanced Parkinson's disease, providing better symptomatic management and enhanced quality of life.
2. D.B.S. is a viable economic alternative to drug therapy.
3. Steps should be taken to ensure that there is equity in queuing for therapy.

ACKNOWLEDGEMENTS

The preparation of this presentation was assisted by an unrestricted educational grant from Medtronic of Canada Ltd. and by The Parkinson Foundation of Canada

APPENDIX B

Reflections on Therapy for Parkinson's Disease

REFLECTIONS ON THERAPY FOR PARKINSON'S DISEASE: MEDICATION AND NEUROSURGERY

BY BILL HARSHAW

Parkinson's disease is associated with free radicals which in turn are associated with the deposition of iron. The human brain is encased in fat. For a person with Parkinson's, the brain, which is the source of the highest creativity and reasoning, spoils and rusts.

The two procedures I had—the pallidotomy in 1993 and the deep brain stimulation the following year—are much in the news as people with Parkinson's (PWPs) search out possible ways to mitigate their symptoms and improve the quality of their lives. Media accounts of these procedures focus on the successes, sometimes spectacular, and give less coverage to the patients whose lives have not increased in quality.

Neurosurgery as a therapy for Parkinson's patients has, with the exception of fetal transplants, passed the point of being experimental. Pallidotomy, Thalamotomy, Deep Brain Stimulation and fetal transplants haven't yet reached the status of bypass surgery for cardiac patients—the gold standard. But it is useful to remember that they are all based on what the noted American physician Lewis Thomas calls "halfway technologies." He does not use this term derisively, but to point out that they do not represent a cure, only better symptom management.

Deep Brain Stimulation appears to be the most effective and economic procedure even though the up-front cost, including the cost of the hardware, makes it more expensive initially.

Neurosurgery for Parkinson's disease has been shown to be effective, efficacious and an improved use of scarce economic resources.

Fetal transplant surgery is to the doctors an extension of the current "gold standard" of treatment, "dopamine replacement therapy," as represented by the L-dopa based medications. However, it has to be shown to be a safe and effective procedure and has a number of ethical and moral hurdles to clear before it becomes acceptable to society generally.

The other procedures fall into the general category of what surgeons do best: "if its broke, fix it" (with apologies to Bert Lance).

To put neurosurgery in the context of the universe of treatment for Parkinson's, it is important to remember that pallidotomy and thalamotomy have been around for fifty years. They were the therapyof choice for advanced PWPs. until the mid 1960s when L-dopa was discovered to be efficacious. As L-dopa gained acceptance, its superiority to all other drug therapies became apparent. Neurosurgery went into eclipse, not to have a renaissance for a quarter century. This period saw the development of a new type of drug—dopamine agonists—that increases and prolong the effectiveness of L-dopa.

A quarter century's use of L-dopa as the medication of choice demonstrated its superiority in symptom management; it also revealed the drug's shortcomings—dyskinesia and psychiatric side effects in advanced patients who were on high doses. In the early1990s, technological advances, the miniaturization of surgical instruments and the need to provide some sort of relief to advanced patients led to a renewal of interest in neurosurgery—the old operations being done more successfully and with greater precision and the invention of Deep Brain Stimulation (DBS). Almost paralleling the surgery was the development of new, non-ergot agonists that, if they live up to their press releases, will provide a meaningful advance on current drug therapy.

Fetal transplantation is considered separately. As a class of surgery, it belongs with organ transplants—heart, lungs, kidney ... the list goes on. It first showed its face in the late 1970s and has been developing quickly since then. At times the pace of progress seems slow to patients, but the rate of change of progress has been nothing short of exponential.

Results of a recent double blind study of fetal transplants[20] were not as good as were expected and are inferior to the results of other types of surgery. About one-third of fetal transplant patients develop severe and disabling dyskinesias—toxic overdoses of dopamine—that appear to be caused by the transplants. The actual mechanism is not clear, but research should shed light on the process causing dyskinesia. Until the causative factors of these dyskinesias are understood, the transplant procedures are likely to receive little positive attention.

Comparing the state of therapy for Parkinson's today to what it was a mere quarter-century ago, the progress is staggering. Before L- dopa, the medications available were a variety of drugs that were serendipitously found to be beneficial as therapy. They were really pretty primitive. Now, there is L-dopa, two generations of agonists, neurosurgery, and a whole new array of research projects, any one of which has the potential to advance treatment markedly. It should be noted that every therapy has its drawbacks, called side effects, which range from the trivial to the serious. Some of these side effects are major enough to prevent certain patients from using some therapies.

Indeed, there is a website on the Internet devoted to patient accounts. The implications of these advances on a broad field of new and newly adapted drug and surgical therapies is that physicians will have several arrows in their quiver when presented with a patient with symptoms that previously would have been intractable. The other aspect is the hope that these developments engender. The American philosopher John Searle noted in a 1995 article:

> As far as we know the relevant processes take place at the micro levels of synapses, neurons, and cell assemblies. All our conscious life is caused by these lower level processes, but we have only the foggiest idea of how it all works.

The doctors know that lesioning works and that chronic stimulation works, yet they do not know how or why. That should give some cause for pause. The same comment can be made, to a degree, with respect to drug therapy. We don't know why some drugs are more effective than others.

Perhaps Parkinson's disease will, in the end, be found to be not one condition, but a cluster of conditions with several common characteristics and each one having unique properties that set it apart. The existence of progressive supra-nuclear palsy and multi-system atrophy are two cases in point. That is why it is a very good thing that there are half a dozen agonists on the market and three types of surgery—lesioning, stimulation, and transplant. One agonist or type of surgery may be more effective than others in different varieties of the condition.

Research is also yielding results on discovering the causes of Parkinson's. PD is caused by the death of the cells comprising the substantia nigra that produce dopamine. It is not known what causes the cells to die. The prevalent current hypothesis is the so-called "double hit" theory—which seems to be the case with other neurodegenerative conditions as well—an hereditary or genetic predisposition that can be hit by an environmental toxin, thus providing the double hit. The toxin could be anything from pesticide and fertilizer to industrial pollutants and smog—it is not known yet. This aspect has caused researchers to investigate the concept of neuroprotection(i.e. what could protect the brain from degeneration?).

Also, as we do not know what causes cell death in the substantia nigra, we do not know whether or not the disease mechanism mutates over time. For instance, were the men Christ cured of the "shaking palsy" in Matthew's Gospel PWPs? If they were, was their PD the same as mine? The answer may well be: "In the main, yes, but there are some important differences." The differences could perhaps arise from the nature of the environmental toxins (assuming the validity of the "double hit" theory)—PCBs weren't around in Biblical times, for example.

This is the fundamental question in neuroscience: what causes cell death and what is the mechanism involved? This question is relevant for multiple sclerosis, ALS, and others.

Relatively few of these procedures have been performed—likely not more than ten thousand in total. There are only about one hundred neurosurgeons in the world who are qualified to perform these procedures. In the context of five million PWPs worldwide, it amounts to a mere fifth of 1 percent. The spectacular results that neurosurgeons have achieved with, it must be added, the help of the patients, are a testament to innovation, imagination and modern technology. The problem is that there are not enough neurosurgeons to satisfy the demand for procedures. In a perfect market, more surgeons would elect functional neurosurgery as a subspecialty until demand and supply was in balance. Alternatively, the fee charged for the procedures could rise until it choked off demand. But, we do not live in a perfect world with only Adam Smith's "invisible hand" to guide us. The marketplace is littered with imperfections ranging from the government and physicians' regulatory bodies to competition amongst surgical specialties.

I am exceedingly fortunate to have had such successful surgeries and had the leading neurosurgeons in this sub-specialty perform them. Others have not been so providential. There is an old aphorism attributed to Abraham Lincoln. The skills of an army general were being recounted to him. When the speaker had concluded, Lincoln responded: "Yes, but is he lucky?". It is not known what the reply was.

I would say that luck goes to the well-prepared. There are numerous anecdotal accounts circulating about patients who have had unfortunate surgical results. To the extent that these histories are accurately reported, they would appear to be the result of one or more of the following factors:

1. The patients may not have been suitable for this type of surgery.
2. The attending physicians and surgeons may not have been adequately qualified, and that standard is very high indeed.
3. The patient and/or his caregiver may have had unrealistic expectations.

Considerations like age (the younger the better), absence of complicating conditions (blood clotting problems, cognitive problems, diabetes, history of stroke or other cerebro-vascular disease), and patient attitude are all important to the medical team in making their decision on whether or not to operate. Patient stamina also plays an important role because of the interactive nature of the procedures—the dialogue between patient and neurosurgeon that is so essential to success. Finally, the neurosurgeon must have an empathetic relationship with the patient because responses to stimuli vary from patient to patient; understanding those differences is crucial.

The public policy implications of the expanded armory now in the hands of the medical profession fall under two headings:

1. young onset Parkinsonians (under 50 years of age), estimated to be 20 percent of all PWPs and

2. late onset, the balance.

The vast majority of young PWPs are in their fifth decade and are likely at or entering their period of peak earning power. If they are denied access to the new drug or surgical therapies through shortage of qualified neurosurgeons, bureaucratic delays in getting drugs approved and on the formulary, this denial would likely cost society money as these individuals might have to go on early retirement or long-term disability. Contributions to social programs would decline as would tax revenue.

Late onset PWPs would face institutional incarceration at no small cost to society.

These comments make no reference to quality of life or the increasing share of the population over 60. Indeed Lang and Lozano point out in their New England Journal of Medicine article that neurodegenerative diseases will surpass cancer as the number two killer by 2040. It makes sense, then, to expedite the approval of new drug therapies and fund additional neurosurgeons from both an economic and a compassionate viewpoint; rarely are these positions synchronous. When they are, it is best to investigate them closely to insure nothing has been missed. To cite my situation anecdotally, my annual drug cost has declined by $10,000 since my DBS five years ago—that has a net present value of $46,500 without considering the cost of long-term care—likely a net present value of least $23,500 for the same time frame, for a total saving of $70,000 before quality of life considerations.

But, this is just my experience.

ENDNOTES

[1] Gwyn, Sandra *Tapestry of War* (Toronto, Harper Collins, 992), p.2

[2] Raines, Howell: *Fly Fishing Through the Midlife Crisis* (New York, William Morrow, 1993)

[3] MacLeish, Archibald: *J.B.* (Boston, Houghton Mifflin, 1958), p.11

[4] Reproductions of coins made without the intention to deceive. They are all stamped "R" on the rim to identify them as such. They would typically be owned by collectors who either could not afford or had not found an original coin of suitable quality.

[5] Oliver Sacks, Wachtel interview

[6] The quotations are from "An Interview with Oliver Sacks" by Eleanor Wachtel in *Brick,* number 50

[7] I wanted to have a good record of the whole procedure, and Pete Paterson was willing to take before, during and after, photographs. The photos accompanying in this book were taken by Peter except for those taken inside the operating room - the hospital medicrats would not allow Peter inside the OR and those pictures were taken by hospital photographers.

[8] New York Review of Books, Vol. 42, #17, p.60

[9] Bill Harshaw is Special Advisor to The Chair of The Parkinson Foundation of Canada. He has spoken and written widely on Parkinson's disease and related issues. Unless otherwise indicated, all quotations in this article ore from his memoir *My Second Life: a memoir of my experience with Parkinson's Disease.*

[10] Sacks, Oliver: *A Leg to Stand On* (New York, Knopf, 198?) p.??

[11] Cather, Willa: *Death Comes for the Archbishop* (New York, Random House, 1992), p.50

[12] C. David Naylor.....

[13] A 'double blind' study is on in which neither the patient nor the rater know which of the therapies the patient is receiving.

[14] The patient's daily prescription medication regime was 2800mg of Sinemet CR 200/50 and 9mg of Permax 1mg daily. He arranged for a three month prescription to save on dispensing fees and negotiated a 10% discount off the drug price. His annual bill for prescription medications was over C$16,000 The savings amounted to over $1,500 annually.

[15] Some readers may be familiar with the concept, popularized in Thomas Costain's novel *The*

Tontine in which the last person alive wins the pool.

[16] Mann, Thomas: "The Making of *The Magic Mountain* in *The Magic Mountain,* p.727

[17] Eliot, T.S.: *Murder in the Cathedral* (London, Faber and Faber, 1935) pp.19f

[18] Alter, David A., Naylor, C. David, Austin, Peter and Tu, Jack V: "Effects of Socioeconomic Status on Access to Invasive Cardiac Procedures and on Mortality after Acute Myocardial Infarction" in *New England Journal of Medicine,* vol. 342, No. 18, pp.1359-67 and Alter, David A., Basinski, Antoni S. and Naylor, C. David: "A Survey of Provider Experiences and Perceptions of Preferential Access to Cardiovascular Care in Ontario, Canada" in *Annals of Internal Medicine* Vol. 159, pp.567-72

[19] Alter, David A., private conversation, October 6, 2000

[20] In this double-blind trial, the control group of patients actually had a mock-surgery, up to and including the drilling of burr holes through the skull and inserting the ultra-fine surgical syringes in the brain. The control group receive nothing further, the test group got fetal mesenchelphic cells. The author knows two participants in this study, one of whom was in

the control group and the other in the test group.

ACKNOWLEDGEMENTS

Bill Harshaw takes pleasure in acknowledging the assistance of the following individuals in the preparation of this presentation:

Dr. David A. Alter, The Institute for Clinical Evaluative Sciences and Sunnybrook Health Sciences Centre, Toronto

Mrs. Jan Duff, R.N. Clinical Trials Manager, Cromedica, Inc., Mississauga

Dr. Anthony F. Graham, Staff Cardiologist, St. Michael's Hospital, Toronto

Dr. Murray Krahn, Assistant Professor, Faculty of Medicine, The University of Toronto

Dr. Antony E. Lang, Director, The Morton and Gloria Shulman Movement Disorders Centre, Toronto Western Hospital and The Jack Clark Professor of Parkinson's Disease Research, The University of Toronto

Dr. Andres M. Lozano, Staff Neurosurgeon, The Toronto Western Hospital and The Ron Tasker Professor of Restorative Neurosurgery, The University of Toronto

Dr. C. David Naylor, Dean of The Faculty of Medicine, The University of Toronto

Pete Paterson is one of Canada's leading photographers. His pictures have appeared in many books and magazines. Pete's studio is in downtown Toronto.

C. David Naylor earned his medical degree from the University of Toronto and was a Rhodes Scholar. At Oxford, he earned a D. Phil. in social and administrative studies. Dr. Naylor is currently Dean of the Faculty of Medicine at the University of Toronto.

Made in the USA
Las Vegas, NV
12 April 2026

45265173R00162